DI·ET DRA·MA \DAHY-it DRAH-muh\

noun

1. Seeing this disguised as a basic math problem when it's actually harder to solve than trigonometry without a calculator:

   > Energy in > Energy out = Our bodies gain weight
   > Energy in < Energy out = Our bodies lose weight
   > Energy in = Energy out = Our bodies stay the same weight

   DISCARD

   Like, are you serious? What is energy? Where does it come from and how does it get in and out of me? What happened to calories? And how do I solve the puzzle when I don't know which equation is right for my body? Argh!

2. Realizing you were supposed to learn the above information in school but didn't, even though you're an honors student.

3. Putting on your favorite outfit and proudly posing for a zillion pictures and posting them on Facebook, only to have the first comment be a snarky one about your size. From your crush.

4. Hearing about the rise in obesity, you decide to start exercising and watching what you eat, until the next day, when the big news is all about how anorexia and bulimia are *also* on the rise, so you vow not to worry *too* much about your body. Until *another* study shows up that causes you to lose your appetite entirely. But not in that way…

5. Worrying you'll be asked to join the next *Teen Mom* cast because you think your gut makes you look preggo.

6. What this book's all about.

(BTW, does this cover make my name look wide?)

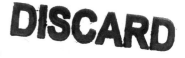

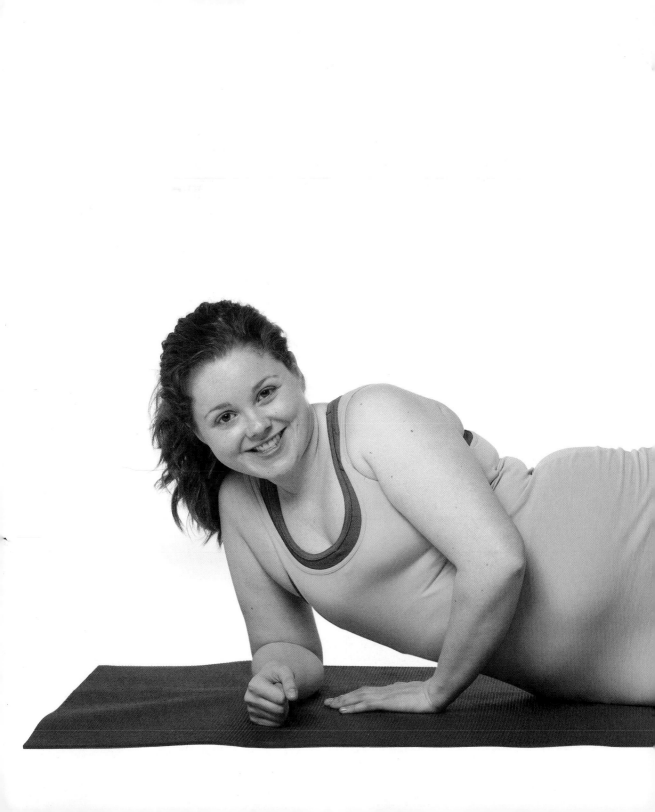

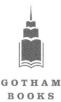

GOTHAM
BOOKS

DIET DRAMA

by Nancy Redd

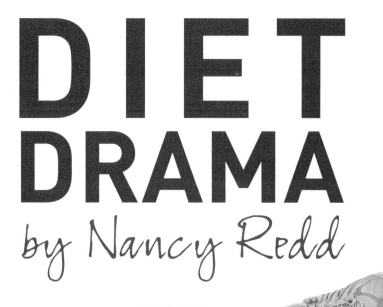

Foreword by Ellen Rome, M.D., M.P.H.
Head of Adolescent Medicine at the Cleveland Clinic

Photography by Kelly Kline and Katy Bea Martinez-Arizala Keller

GOTHAM BOOKS
Published by Penguin Group (USA) Inc.
375 Hudson Street, New York, New York 10014, U.S.A.
Penguin Group (Canada), 90 Eglinton Avenue East, Suite 700, Toronto, Ontario M4P 2Y3, Canada
(a division of Pearson Penguin Canada Inc.); Penguin Books Ltd, 80 Strand, London WC2R 0RL,
England; Penguin Ireland, 25 St Stephen's Green, Dublin 2, Ireland (a division of Penguin Books Ltd);
Penguin Group (Australia), 250 Camberwell Road, Camberwell, Victoria 3124, Australia (a division of
Pearson Australia Group Pty Ltd); Penguin Books India Pvt Ltd, 11 Community Centre, Panchsheel
Park, New Delhi—110 017, India; Penguin Group (NZ), 67 Apollo Drive, Rosedale, North Shore
0632, New Zealand (a division of Pearson New Zealand Ltd); Penguin Books (South Africa) (Pty) Ltd,
24 Sturdee Avenue, Rosebank, Johannesburg 2196, South Africa

Penguin Books Ltd, Registered Offices: 80 Strand, London WC2R 0RL, England

Published by Gotham Books, a member of Penguin Group (USA) Inc.

First printing, December 2010
10 9 8 7 6 5 4 3 2 1

Gotham Books and the skyscraper logo are trademarks of Penguin Group (USA) Inc.

Cataloging-in-Publication Data is available at the Library of Congress

ISBN 978-1-592-40602-9
Printed in the United States of America

Producer and Creative Director: Nancy Redd
nancy@nancyredd.com
www.nancyredd.com

While the author has made every effort to provide accurate telephone numbers and Internet addresses at
the time of publication, neither the publisher nor the author assumes any responsibility for errors, or for
changes that occur after publication. Further, the publisher does not have any control over and does not
assume any responsibility for author or third-party Web sites or their content.

PUBLISHER'S NOTE: Neither the publisher nor the author is engaged in rendering professional advice
or services to the individual reader. The ideas, procedures, and suggestions contained in this book
are not intended as a substitute for consulting with your physician or health professional. All matters
regarding your health require medical supervision. Neither the author nor the publisher shall be liable
or responsible for any loss or damage allegedly arising from any information or suggestion in this book.

To my incredible mother, Mrs. Amanda H. Redd,
for her catchy and endless encouragement, optimism, support, and love.
Thanks for teaching me how to look my best at all sizes!

And to my beyond awesome big brother, Sammy Redd Jr.,
for refusing to let me be lazy when it came to exercising my brain.
I am a lucky little sister!

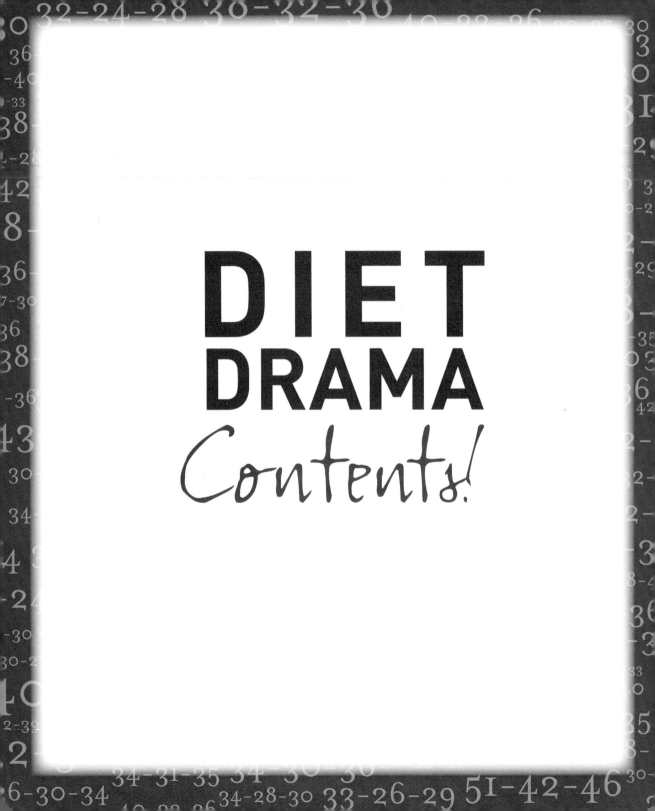

DIET
DRAMA
Contents!

LOVE *Your Body!*

MOVE Your Body!

FEED *Your Body!*

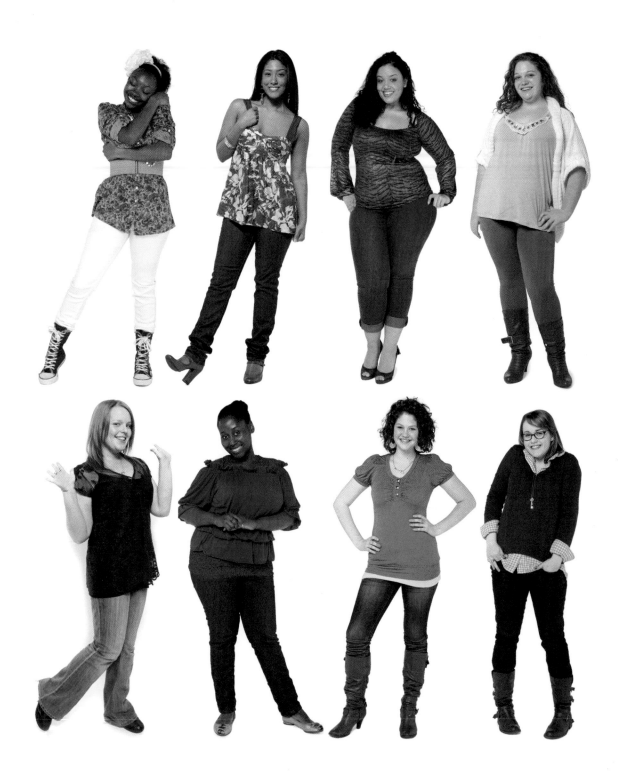

FOREWORD

ELLEN ROME, M.D., M.P.H.
Head of Adolescent Medicine at the Cleveland Clinic

Girls today have it rough! The media sends kids mixed messages, simultaneously promoting products and foods that encourage excess in everyday life, while glamorizing dangerously-thin models and celebrities as the "picture of health." This has left most teens without a clue as to how to build and maintain a healthy body. Many don't even know the range of what a healthy body actually looks like and struggle to comprehend that striving for a size zero is not the same as striving for health! "I'm fat" is a common refrain in my clinic, whether the girl actually has excess body fat or not. The emotional pressure on today's teens is tremendous and troubling.

Quite often, however, my patients truly are in need of better eating and exercise habits, and at the Cleveland Clinic, we're always ready to help. We're devoted to turning the tide of pediatric obesity, and most importantly, we're accomplishing realistic and long-lasting individual, family, and community change with no "thin" obsession or "heavy" discrimination. Shame, guilt, and blame have no place in the health and wellness field — wherever an individual begins their path to wellness, and however slowly they might go, they deserve to be treated with respect, dignity, and kindness. What we're doing is working. In just a few short years, with a lot of hard work, Cleveland has moved from one of the "25 Fattest Cities in America" to one of the top "15 *Fittest* Cities in America." We could have opted for a quick, flashy fix: "Let's put our city on a diet!" but we knew that we wanted long-term results, and that diets don't work for whole cities any better than they do on an individual basis.

We offer teens a unique, state-of-the-art, personable approach that encourages health at every step of the journey, and I am proud of that, but I am also worried for the rest of our country. Even though excess body fat is primed to surpass smoking as the number one preventable cause of death in America, medical professionals are often unprepared to treat the growing number of overweight and obese youth not just physically but also psychologically.

Mainstream diet books aimed at teens aren't much better, as they are often just restrictive mini-versions of adult plans that aren't adjusted for the needs of the adolescent body. When looking for source materials and product recommendations to encourage and educate these girls as well as for other health professionals, I found little out there that was worth sharing. For example, the adolescent brain requires 30-50 grams of fat daily for proper brain development. Thus, diet books that suggest a limited fat intake, though popular in the adult crowd, are inappropriate and unhealthy for teens. Also, as any parent or teacher can attest, adolescents are extremely sensitive and require extensive encouragement and assistance in building and preserving self-esteem, and the age-appropriate diet literature commonly available lacks this important step. Until now.

Now, I can recommend something positive and inspiring. *Diet Drama* provides a refreshing, frank take on how to encourage teen girls to do their best to be healthy for life and for the right reasons. Teens don't need fad diets ever, and few require weight loss surgery if given the right tools early enough. These tools include emotional support, plus basic health and nutrition information ideally taught to the child from toddlerhood through adolescence. Unfortunately, today's teens are rarely given the basic health tools needed to make sensible, consistent choices of what to eat, how much to eat, and when to eat. Adolescents spend most of their free time sitting at the computer, texting, or watching television, and processed foods have shifted from tasty treats on rare occasions to daily fare, with large numbers of teens eating fast food for at least one meal per day. This inactivity and lack of healthy nutrition has caused girls to start seeing me and my staff with diseases previously reserved only for adults: type 2 diabetes, high blood pressure, knee and lower back pain from excess weight, and other disturbing health challenges. Nancy always says that "no body is perfect," and I share her belief, but we both agree that everybody has the right to enjoy good health physically and emotionally.

Diet Drama fills a huge hole in the health world—with the goal of making more girls whole! Whether the reader is looking for help because she's obese, overweight, trying to tone up, or just wants to maintain her healthy body, she doesn't need a sixty-day diet plan; she needs a *lifetime* plan expressed in easy-to-understand language with practical strategies. Teen girls need help detaching from the messages of the billion-dollar diet industry, which seductively promotes the latest expensive meal plans and disordered eating practices. This book is the first to combine understandable, accessible language with medically accurate information in a manner that is pithy, practical, and a powerful tool for change.

In *Diet Drama*, Nancy honestly and sympathetically gives girls a courageous and important reality check on body-related issues along with clear, entertaining, medically accurate information, candid confessions about her own painful experiences and struggles, self-esteem-boosting tips and tricks, and photos of real girls' bodies without the "benefits" of airbrushing. No body is perfect, indeed, but this book is as close as it gets! *Diet Drama* is an easy-to-understand, inclusive guide for girls of all body types, sizes, and motivation levels that speaks to today's teens with positive, helpful guidance. This book is a great gift for girls around the globe who need to know how to talk about and take care of their bodies without bashing themselves or feeling ashamed. Having seen Nancy in action with her first book, *Body Drama*, I believe she's a pitch-perfect role model for what today's teens need to hear about health, weight, and body image. Whether you're a parent, a health professional, or a pre-teen or teen, read it, share it, laugh with it, and celebrate the ways girls can succeed at getting in shape without resorting to dangerous diet drama!

If Your Doctor Has You on a "Diet"

f.y.i.

So, if "diet" is a dirty word, what should you do if a professional has put you on a diet? Well, if you're one of the lucky few who is working very closely with a nutritionist, dietician, clinician, doctor, or other medical expert who is carefully supervising what you eat and how you exercise, with frequent check-ins, adjustments, and follow-ups, that's great! You've got a trusted person who knows what they're talking about to help you create an effective, long-term game plan for getting healthy and achieving your specific goals. However, if your doctor has simply suggested (or demanded) that you go on a diet without offering any one-on-one long-term help, take it upon yourself to substitute the word "diet" for "move your body" and "feed your body" so that you can focus on something more than just losing a few pounds, like a lifetime of health and happiness!

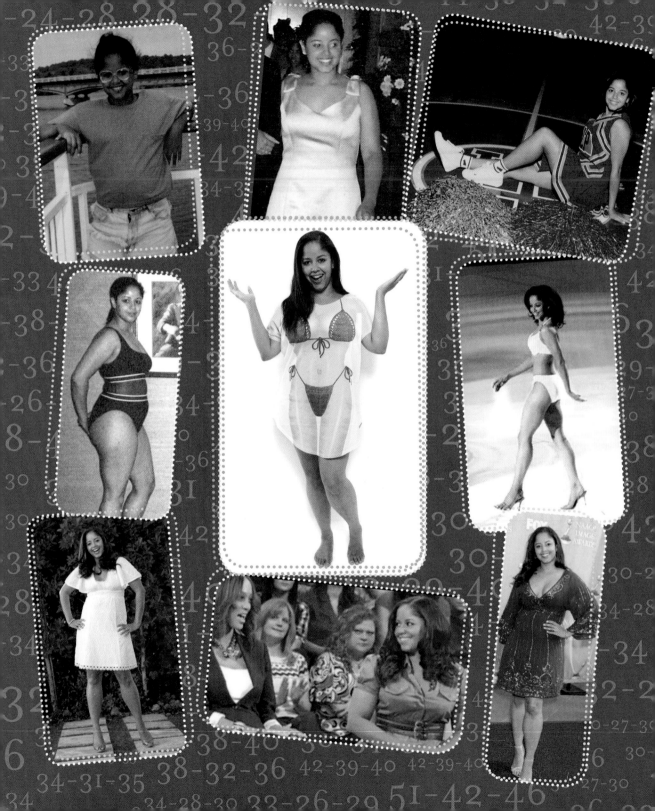

INTRODUCTION
NANCY REDD
Author

I've said it once, and I'll say it again: No body's perfect! You're probably used to diet books screaming scary statistics about obesity and anorexia to threaten you into eating right and exercising regularly, right? Well not here! If you're anything like I am, and a lot of you are, guilt and shame won't lower the numbers on your scale, and fear won't build better food habits. I've been a stressed-out size double-zero (when I won the Miss America swimsuit competition) and a totally confident size twelve (when I won $250,000 on *Who Wants to be a Millionaire?*), but I've also felt bad about myself while at high weights, and felt great while at low weights, too. After losing and regaining the same fifty pounds repeatedly and emptying my pockets on products that don't work, you know what I've learned? Diets don't work, especially in the long run. In fact, teen girls who diet

◄·········· that's me!

using strict food plans gain more weight than those who *don't* diet! Why? The pressure a "diet" puts on us to eat perfectly and exercise to exhaustion causes binges and unhealthy eating habits during diet breaks, creating an evil, expensive cycle of frustration and self-hate.

The U.S. diet industry, which earns 60 *billion* dollars each year, knows how to tap into our insecurities in order to sell products. We spend our cash on countless diet plans, some of them dangerous, that blame and fault us girls, making us believe that any size over a two will keep us from being healthy, fitting in, finding love, and feeling worthy. But that's not true! It's commonly thought that losing weight—and lots of it—always leads to gaining self-esteem, but think again! Women with extra body fat are not the only ones who start dangerous diets, undertake intense exercise routines, or crave plastic surgery. Girls of all shapes and sizes are dissatisfied and uncomfortable with themselves because it seems like we could always be just a little thinner, trimmer, and more toned. This alone is enough to make us give up before even getting started — nothing is ever good enough!

I've yo-yoed and had body drama at all sizes, and I've been teased and tormented by others while also bashing my own body behind closed doors. You know what I've learned? That getting healthy and being happy in your own skin has less to do with your size than your mind. Inside this book I talk candidly about my own journey because I want to help you start figuring out how to feel good *emotionally* about your body at all times—not just when you have reached your physical goal at the end of a diet, but throughout your entire life at all sizes and weights.

I won't be winning another bikini contest anytime soon, and today, as a curvy size eight (sometimes a ten or a twelve), I'm not slender like most diet book authors, but what I've written here works for me! Although I sometimes slim down (perhaps for a big party) and sometimes put on a few pounds (when I'm stressed out, see page 241), I have stayed around a healthy range for my build and height for the past five years without the "help" of any expensive fad diets that would have eventually failed. Most importantly, regardless of my dress size, I feel good about myself at all times—not just when I fit into my skinny jeans. I eat better than I did when I was very thin, and I am far more active now than I was when exercise was reserved for those few times a year when I crash dieted. I am strong, grounded, and in love with myself and with someone else, and we both adore my body independent of my clothing size. It's so fun and empowering to live this way, and you too can find your healthy range and stay there without suffering through stupid diets!

To help you ditch your diet drama, I decided to write another body book that starts from scratch. Believe me, I know that you worry about your weight not just because you want to fit into your jeans but also because you want to fit in with your friends! That's why *Diet Drama* is the first book of its kind that not only builds a foundation of basic body smarts when it comes to food and fitness but that also shares personal stories and common scenarios about the related issues of body image, self-esteem, and stress. Let's face it: Many of us are never formally taught how to eat right and exercise. It's all too easy to fall for fad diets when we're unhappy with our bodies and want to do something about it, because we don't know any other way to get in shape! At any given time, 41 percent of Americans are on a diet with an average weight-loss goal of thirty-seven pounds. But incredibly, five years *after* their diets end, 95 percent of dieters end up heavier than they were before they started! That's because for most of us, it's impossible to go from couch potato to celebrity look-a-like in six weeks, no matter how many products we purchase that promise just that.

I'm no stranger to wanting to believe these bogus claims, and I've been let down by a lot of books and programs that did me more harm than good. It's no wonder that most of us have unreasonable expectations of our bodies when even honors students make it through school without learning the nutrition and exercise basics that are essential to health! (I have e-mails from *Body Drama* readers to prove it.) *Diet Drama* is here to fill in the health holes that cause confusion and can make all the difference when you are trying to get in shape. Say, for example, that you are exercising regularly and growing fitter and you could swear your body looks slimmer, but you get on the scale only to find that your weight has gone *up*. What? You expected it to go *down*! Should you cry? No. Should you give up and gobble an entire German chocolate cake in self pity? NO! The culprit is not your body or your exercise efforts. It's misinformation! This exact scenario happened to me in high school, and if I had known the basics, that muscle weighs more than fat, and that instead of stressing over the number on the scale I should have checked my measurements or paid attention to the fit of my clothes, I wouldn't have turned to an entire batch of chocolate-chip cookies for comfort!

From super-simple visuals showing proper portion sizes, to how to deal with fat-talking friends, to exercises that are easy to do anywhere, anytime, *Diet Drama* is packed with powerful, easy-to-understand, and entertaining information to help you stop stressing out and start seeing yourself—and your health—as more than just your size. "Thin" might be in, but a low number on the scale isn't the healthiest—or the most realistic—goal for everyone. So instead of promoting the myths that one body type, diet plan, or exercise routine is the best, *Diet Drama* is here to help you break the cycle of shame and stress so that you can look and feel your personal best, whether you are a size two, twelve, or twenty-two.

This might not be the first diet book you've ever read, but I bet that it's the last one you'll ever need!

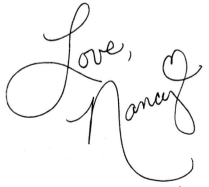

Love,
Nancy

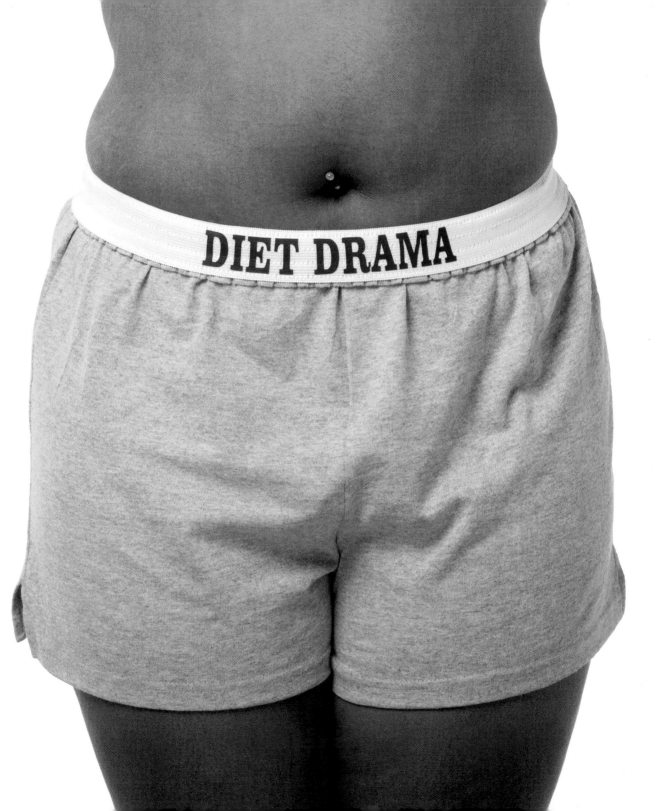

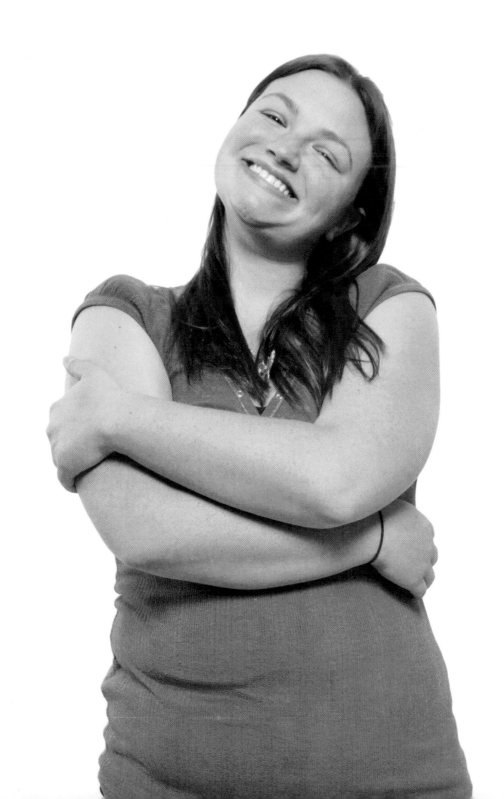

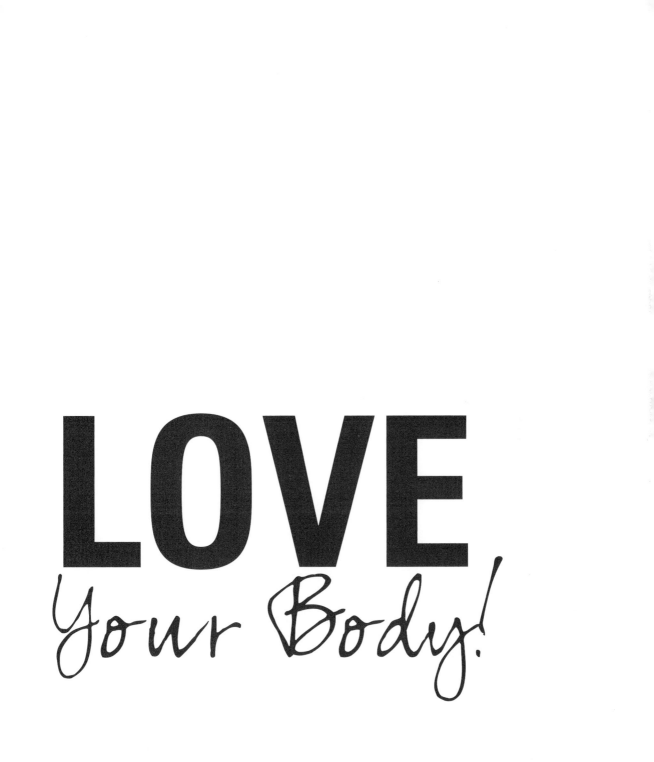

"Nancy, take that fat suit off!" My heart stopped as soon as my friend Jen's words hit my ears, and I immediately pressed the pause button to stop the video of me winning $250,000 on *Who Wants to Be a Millionaire?* Did she say what I thought she said? Before I could respond, Jen, while still staring at the 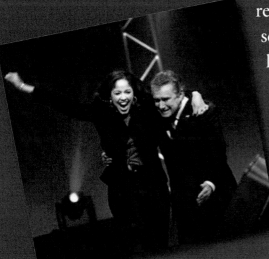 screen, excitedly exclaimed, "Wow, you look sooooo much better now!" Sure, Jen didn't know me back when I was a few sizes heavier, but that show was one of my proudest moments, and I thought I looked really good in the hot seat! Embarrassed, I immediately changed the topic—and the tape— and we went back to studying.

In an instant and with only six words, my biggest source of pride became my most humiliating moment. After that, I worried that everyone who saw me on the show thought that I was fat. Whenever friends excitedly told me that they caught a rerun of me with Regis, I worried that they, too, were thinking what only Jen had the nerve to say. For a long time,

Learning how to love your body is perhaps the most difficult of no matter what I weighed, I beat myself up about my body on a daily basis, convincing myself that I was ugly and gross, and that everything needed improvement before I could ever be happy with myself. Can you relate?

Learning how to love your body is perhaps the most difficult of all diet dramas when it comes to getting and staying healthy. That's why I'm starting *Diet Drama* with this chapter, because no amount of healthy eating and exercise can completely reverse a bad body image. Before tackling health-oriented habits, we need to realize how shameful feelings and negative talk about our bodies affect us, our relationships with others, and our dreams for ourselves.

Years passed before I was able to look at myself on *Millionaire* without a cringe-worthy "Nancy, take that fat suit off!" ringing in my ears. Today I still think of Jen when the topic comes up, but enough time has passed that I now have a healthier reaction to her cruel comment. I no longer take her words to heart, and I just think of the experience as one of many times when my personal concept of beauty was challenged. I had to work hard to remind myself that for every person like Jen who might make hateful comments, I received dozens of e-mails congratulating me and complimenting me on

all diet dramas when it comes to getting and staying healthy!

fast fact

Girls and women who read fashion magazines are much more critical of their own bodies than those who do not read fashion magazines.

fast fact

Experts estimate that only ONE in every one hundred women naturally possess the current "ideal" face shape, skin color, and body type favored by the media and, usually, ourselves: Caucasian, tall, very thin (but with large breasts), and symmetrical features. The rest of us are left out. No wonder staring in the mirror is stressful. We are comparing ourselves to someone it is physically impossible to look like!

my appearance on the show. Instead of seeing myself on screen in a "fat suit," I finally started to again see myself in my favorite earrings, with a nice hairstyle, and holding a hefty check I'd earned by using my brain!

It's impossible to control the actions of others, so instead of worrying about what the people around you consider attractive and desirable, it's time to learn to live life for yourself! I wish that I had told Jen how her words made me feel instead of keeping my reaction inside. (I guess she knows now!) But I admit that what she said shouldn't have mattered so much. The super-slim, perky-breasted, cellulite-free beauty ideals endorsed by magazines and television make it easier for others to compare and judge us (more on this on page 27), but often *we* are our own toughest critics, allowing our mismatched beauty ideals to control how we see ourselves.

While it's easy to be your own worst enemy when it comes to body

While that comment from Jen sparked a battle in my brain about my attractiveness and self-worth, I'm proud to say that I'm now winning the war against body bashing. Nowadays I control how I allow myself to feel and think about my body. I never ever talk terribly about my body or anyone else's, even if she's a celebrity and can't hear me. No one—I repeat, no one—deserves body bashing! Stopping the fat talk and body bashing is hard at first, but let me tell you, it feels great to speak nothing but good about your body and everybody else's!

This chapter will help you learn how to handle negative people, but more important, it will help you learn how to handle yourself. While it's easy to be your own worst enemy when it comes to body image and emotions, it's much better to become your own best friend. Remember, no matter how often others judge you or how often you judge yourself, no referees or rules govern body image. The only person who can call a foul or come up with the final verdict is you. So please read this chapter first, and reread it often to make sure that you're prepared to make the right call!

image and emotions, it's much better to become your own best friend!

WHAT DOES IT MEAN TO LOVE *My Body?*

Loving your body starts with having a good body image, which is how you see yourself in relation to your personal beauty ideal. Whether we know it or not, each of us has a beauty ideal. Want to figure out yours? Close your eyes and picture the perfect female your age from head to toe. Does she have lots of junk in her trunk? Freckles? Hazel eyes? A tiny waist? A flat chest? Red hair? Dimples on her cheeks? Dimples on her butt? That perfect girl as you just imagined is your beauty ideal. She's the one you rank as #1 in the looks department.

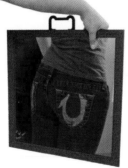

Now be honest: When you thought about your beauty ideal, how much did she resemble you? Did she look exactly like you? Nothing like you? Were some features, such as her hair, face, boobs, height, or butt the same as yours while others were different? How close you are to your beauty ideal affects your body image, which determines how much you love your body, which in turn affects your self-esteem, confidence, happiness, and life in general.

If we all looked exactly the same, we would all probably love our bodies because there wouldn't be a hierarchy of hotness. However, since we all look different, magazines, movies, and other media rank our physical characteristics, and we tend to buy into whatever they tell us to believe. And usually they are telling us that something's wrong with nearly everything about our bodies! What is the #1 characteristic that magazines like to compare and contrast? You guessed it. Women's weight! "Thin is in," and not just slender, but extremely small bodies are "in style" right now. The thinner your body, the better, according to the media, to the point where dangerously underweight celebrities and models are celebrated on magazine covers, with any incremental weight gain being noted—and bashed—in next week's issue. (Extreme thinness hasn't always been the cultural ideal. Turn to page 32 for past beauty ideals!)

The problem is that only a small number of us naturally fit this beauty ideal: thin and (often) large-breasted. The select few who fit that mold become our beauty ideals, as they are photographed, praised, and celebrated solely for their external appearance. But what about the rest of us who aren't naturally very thin? Most of us go one of two ways: Either we crash diet down to an unhealthy weight to be considered hot, or we feel huge and loathe our bodies because a healthy size for our frame is a six or a fourteen, not a double-zero.

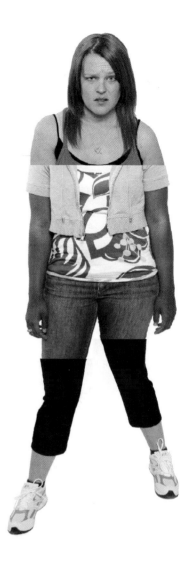

It's tough to ignore what society considers beautiful, and it's hard to resist ranking yourself, whether you think you're at the top or the bottom of the list. In fact, 90 percent of girls feel as if the media puts a *lot* of pressure on them to be thin, causing up to 70 percent of girls who are a healthy weight to consider themselves overweight, and one out of every three to admit to starving themselves to try to lose weight! Those of us not considered beautiful by societal standards often feel as if we're supposed to move aside to make room for the thinner, prettier people. Beauty based on characteristics we cannot control arouses powerful emotions—from shame and embarrassment to depression and anger—causing us to dislike ourselves and our bodies. Size obsession has become so stressful in our society that in a recent survey on self-esteem, only women who were ten pounds *underweight* had a positive body image, even if they were destroying their health to achieve that weight!

Misery in the form of hunger pains and self-hate isn't the only way to deal with impossible beauty ideals. You have another option:

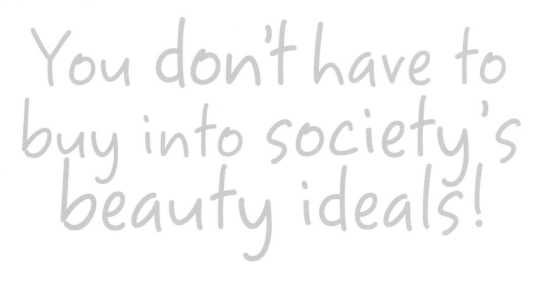

You don't have to buy into society's beauty ideals!

While those ideals might affect how some people treat you (see page 65 for how to deal with body bashers), no one can force you to let media hype affect your mind-set about who you are and what you deserve. Nothing about your self-esteem is set in stone or written in permanent ink, whether or not you need to eat better and exercise more often. Starting today, you can erase everything negative and start writing your own script starring *your* physical features and *your* best self as your personal beauty ideal!

Maybe your beauty ideal features a "better" you that you're working toward healthily, one who happens to have more arm muscles or a tighter tummy. But if when you close your eyes, you see a version of you as your beauty ideal and not someone else's unattainable face and frame, your body image is bound to rebound and you'll be loving your body in no time!

OK, this is so embarrassing, but I had an obsession with a certain celebrity that lasted for years. I coveted everything about her face and body, especially the body parts that were most unlike mine, like her impossibly tiny waist and tight rear, which I praised as much better than my mushy tushy. I even got a (really bad) version of her haircut in high school and bought an (even worse) copy of a dress she wore to the Oscars once for one of my first college formals. I was committed to imitating her, but even at my smallest size, no matter how many crunches I did or how much I dieted, I never came close to matching her figure. When I compared my photographs with hers, I never considered the fact that she had a different body type than I did, nor did I see how hot I looked or how fit I was in my own right, and I never patted myself on the back for all those hours in the gym. All I could see was my failure to accomplish mission impossible.

Today, I look back and think, "How ridiculous!" And I'm angry that I spent so much of my short time as a size zero lamenting over my looks in comparison to a supermodel instead of traipsing around in a string bikini. But at the time, I took myself—and my body's faults (compared to hers)—very seriously, and the entire thing was deeply depressing. When I finally snapped out of it, got sick of my self-pity, and decided to write **Body Drama,** guess what I realized? The only person putting me in competition with a supermodel was me! And the only people putting your body in competition with others is you! None of us have to buy into other people's beauty ideals. We can create our own!

Conveniently, my current beauty ideal looks a lot like me on my very best days, give or take a few pounds (easily shed in a few months by exercising more and eating better) and chin hairs (easily shed in a couple of seconds with a terrific pair of tweezers). For the past few years—and for the first time in my life—I am loving my body more and more each day. The person I see when I look in the mirror today is what I want most to look like tomorrow, and she'll be my beauty ideal for the rest of my life!

29

WHY SHOULD I LOVE *My Body?*

More Than I Love Society's Beauty Ideals?

Some of you might be thinking that loving your own body is common sense, but sadly, many of us are convinced that the lucky few who have won the looks lottery are somehow better than the rest of us! If you've been brainwashed to believe you should worship women that you'll never resemble—if you think that it's OK to be called fat or ugly or to call yourself fat or ugly—you're letting a negative body image affect more than your looks. Not loving your body affects:

✪ how you move your body. When you hate your body, it's common to avoid exercise out of embarrassment (not wanting to be seen in gym clothes) or to exercise constantly for the wrong reasons. Somehow, exercise has gotten a bad rap as something painful and dull only done in an

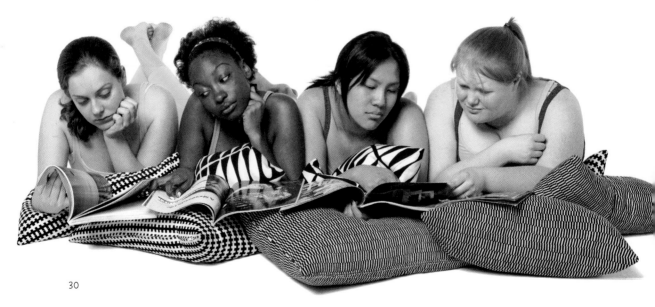

expensive gym or on a boring machine in an effort to create a Barbie-like body. But when you love your body, you don't look at exercise as an evil part of being healthy; you look at being active as a great way to relieve stress, build strength, and feel good! Turn to page 81 to learn how to exercise with a focus on strength and stability rather than a focus on fitting into a size zero!

✮ how you feed your body. All foods are okay to eat in moderation (meaning you shouldn't live off a steady diet of donuts and fries, but having them a few times a month is fine), but when you hate your body, it's easy to get hooked on emotional eating habits, such as eating mostly junk, overeating, or not eating much at all. Turn to page 165 to learn how to eat better and start seeing how great you feel when you fill yourself up with tasty and healthy foods instead of gross garbage that makes you feel bad and look even worse!

✮ what you think you deserve and can accomplish. Not loving your body affects more than your thoughts about your appearance. It can get you down about your entire life! From serious amounts of stress to poor school performance to skipping social activities to rejecting romantic opportunities (or worse, only getting involved with mean people that put you down, like my ex-boyfriend that I tell you about on page 146), hating your body can make you miss out on things because you think that only "perfect" people deserve to feel beautiful, find love, experience success, and enjoy happiness. Don't waste any more time with those terrible thoughts!

Even if you're trying to slim down some, separate your size from your self-worth and see how much happier you become. Women of all shapes and sizes are loved and lead happy, healthy, wonderful lives. So can you if you let yourself break free from a bad body image!

BTW: GUYS HAVE DIET DRAMA, TOO!

The media's excessive focus on big muscles and tiny waists has pushed millions of men into buying diet and muscle-gain products, many of which are as useless— or dangerous!—as the products that are marketed to women. While you might laugh and say, "Finally!" body hate is no healthier in males than it is in females. Discourage the dudes in your life from stressing out about their chest size!

Beauty Ideals Through History

Super-thin wasn't always in. Check out these beauty ideals from back in the day! If some of these figures look a lot like yours, think of your personal beauty ideal as a sign that you're classic, old-school, or retro. Or, consider yourself fashion forward, as everything old eventually becomes new again!

25,000 years ago – The Venus of Willendorf

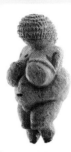

One of the first carvings of the human form, this plump, large-breasted, heavy-hipped beauty ideal wasn't a realistic representation of the women of the time. It was an idealized image, which is a fancy way of saying that many women probably wished they looked like this. Very few, if any, did. (Sound familiar?) My, how times have changed . . . or have they? A different body type was coveted, but with the same impossibility!

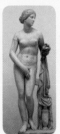

2,400 years ago – Aphrodite of Cnidus

This naked Aphrodite is the oldest large statue of a female nude known in classical sculpture. The artist painstakingly portrayed the goddess of love not as a weak waif but as a healthy woman with a curvy, strong body.

400 years ago – Rubenesque Paintings

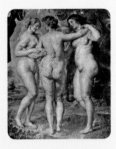

Artist Peter Paul Rubens (1577-1640) was fond of painting full-bodied women. Cellulite, body folds, and tummy rolls were considered beautiful—a worthy focus in artwork—unlike today when such traits are airbrushed away in published photographs. In Rubens's era, extra weight was considered a sign of health and wealth.

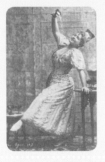

100 years ago – Singer Lillian Russell

With her weight hovering around two hundred pounds, this big-boned Broadway singer was considered the feminine ideal of her generation. Men admired and women envied her full figure. She even had a rose named in her honor: the American Beauty!

HOW CAN I LOVE My Body?

Sometimes it helps to realize that even the models and stars frequently hate their bodies and do not see in themselves what society sees. Although we see them as "perfect," some tiny models torment themselves about every imagined flaw and they may feel as bad about their bodies as the rest of us sometimes do! Many boo-hoo behind closed doors with a bad body image, unable to hold down healthy relationships with people or food. At the same time, many women who are far from what our society considers "beautiful" have a great body image and love their lives! They love their bodies and believe themselves to be total babes, and their romantic partners agree! Wait a minute. What gives?

Loving your body and having a good body image can spring from feeling good inside yourself—feeling good about your body, your health, and your place in this world. While it's true that no one is immune to body angst, ALL of us have the power to take control and create our own beauty ideals that better represent who we are and what we love about our bodies. Advertisements and a culture of body bashing have taught *all* of us to scrutinize our bodies in search of the smallest flaws from the size of a stomach to the length of a toe to the shape of a forehead (True story: I was asked to alter my forehead while I was Miss Virginia; for the details check out page 37.) If your beauty ideals are based on the spoken and unspoken suggestions that come from outside yourself—the people you hang out with, the community you live in, the magazines and books you read, the romantic crushes you have, the movies and television shows you watch—what are you doing? You aren't thinking for yourself. You are merely accepting the opinions of others. And, remember, those suggestions are only *opinions*!

There is an alternative. Just like you don't have to buy into beauty ideals, you don't have to swallow the opinions of others, either! Even if you think there's room for improvement, there's absolutely no reason to hate your body. So stop beating yourself up and start seeing yourself as what you truly are: beautiful just as you are, inside and out!

The process of learning to love your body is not a short or especially easy one, but it all starts when you banish body bashing, stop focusing on weight, and accept the shape mother nature gave you.

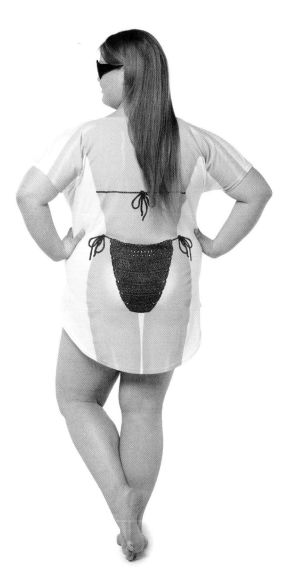

You LOVE Your Body When You...
BANISH BODY BASHING

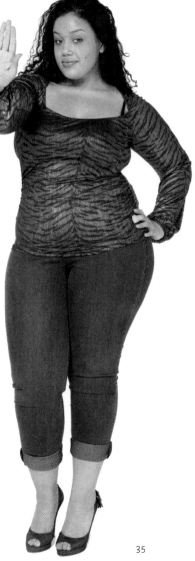

Only 2 percent of women worldwide consider themselves beautiful! And most teens who are actually at a healthy weight don't even believe that they are—only 38 percent of healthy-weight teens think that they are "about the right size," with one in every five considering her body as "too fat." Such distorted views are so widespread that experts have invented the term "normative discontent," which is a fancy way of saying that being content with your body is *unusual* for almost all of us girls!

Because we don't love our bodies, we tend to bash them for everything and anything we can criticize. From whines about weight to critiques on cellulite to nitpicks about our noses, body bashing turns our defenseless, didn't-do-anything-to-us *outsides* into punching bags as we attempt to relieve the anxiety we feel *inside*. Instead of making us feel better, grumbling about our waistlines and complaining about our cankles only makes us feel worse and our "problem areas" seem even more problematic.

When you break free from body bashing—not just your own body but the bodies of others, too—you stop accepting the media's opinions and start thinking for yourself. You start believing that your health and your happiness and giving others the same respect you deserve are what's most important.

WHEN OTHERS BASH YOU

Have you been the victim of bashing? You're not alone! One in four teens are regularly bullied and bashed, with consequences ranging from low self-esteem to depression and suicide. Don't let others' actions and words work your nerves and ruin your life. Turn to the drama on page 65 for tips on how to deal with being bullied and bashed about your body.

STOP BASHING YOURSELF

Have you ever had an annoying kid grab your arm and start hitting you in the face with your own hand, all the while giggling and saying, "Stop hitting yourself! Stop hitting yourself!"? That's a lot like body bashing; you're beating yourself up for no reason! Remember, like I said on page 28, the only person putting you in competition with others is YOU. Think about it . . . if magazines, movies, and television featured models with a couple of inches to pinch, we wouldn't look at our love handles with such hate. If plastic surgeons promoted cellulite *increasing* treatments as this season's must-have, we'd be clipping clothespins onto our thighs to create those in-demand dents! It's all so arbitrary, which is a fancy way of saying random. You do need to strive for health, but you do NOT need to buy into popular beauty ideals!

Even if you agree with what the media calls beautiful, you don't have to bash yourself just because you don't look like a model or a movie star. Society's ideas about health and beauty don't work for many people. Even those with the so-called perfect body still sometimes find themselves body bashing, even when technically there's nothing to bash—it's a horrible habit that you can control! So forget what you see in magazines and movies. Stop body bashing today and start seeing yourself as more than your shape and size.

I CONFESS:

I WAS CONVINCED MY FOREHEAD NEEDED FIXING!

"Nancy, I've gotta tell you something," said my pageant coach when she called me up to chat. After months of preparation for the Miss America Pageant, I was used to being critiqued not only about my size, but also about **everything,** from the color of my elbows (too dark) to the length of my nails (too nubby), but nothing could have prepared me for what she was about to say. "I'm going to come right out and say it: Your forehead is all wrong." My **forehead**? "It's standing out in all your pictures. Your forehead is too low on the sides and it looks like your hairline is trying to mate with your eyebrows. We've gotta do something about it."

At this point, the competition was so close and I was so stressed that short of being battered and fried "to improve texture," I would have done anything. So I gingerly asked, "How do I fix it?"

"Well," she sighed, "it's too late for your pictures. We'll have to airbrush those some more, but I think you should get those patches of hair jutting out of the side of your forehead waxed off ASAP." Ten minutes later and twenty dollars poorer, I was free of an inch of hair on each side of my forehead, and my hairline went from looking like the outline of a naturally occurring puzzle piece to an egg. While I supposedly looked cleaner and fresher, I was disappointed. I thought my face looked a whole lot better before, but I dared not disagree!

Imagine my shock when a few weeks later, a fan stopped me and gasped, "Your thing-a-ma-jigs!" and pointed to my now-bald forehead. "Where'd they go? That's my favorite thing about you. It's so unusual and I wish I had them!"

I immediately cancelled my standing monthly waxing appointment and never looked back, but it shouldn't have taken a total stranger to set me straight on what suited my face. The old saying is right. Beauty is in the eye of the beholder, and you can't let anyone else decide what looks good on you. Stay strong and steer clear of others' opinions!

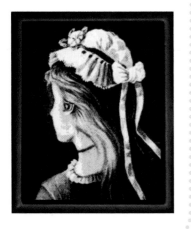
STOP BASHING OTHERS

While you're at it, ban yourself and your friends from bashing not just your own bodies, but other peoples' bodies as well, whether real-life friends and acquaintances or the celebrities in magazines and on television that seem like "fair game" to tease because they're putting themselves out there. Don't be a hip-size hypocrite! The more you bash the bodies of others, the more generally accepted body bashing becomes, and the less you can complain when someone says something mean about you. No one is perfect (we can *all* improve!), but try to identify the problem without pointedly saying something bad about a person's body.

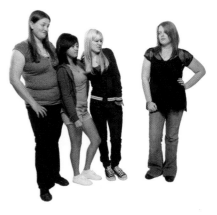

For example, telling your BFF that a model's small size in a certain magazine "is really irresponsible of the company and makes me not want to buy any of their clothes" is a fair statement of your opinion based on facts. It's certainly a big improvement over body bashing her by saying "she's a skinny witch with neck bones so sharp they'd cut you if you tried to hug her!" That kind of statement is hurtful and promotes hate, and you want to spread healthy body love and happiness!

The same thing goes for people you don't like. You may have a legit reason for disliking the girl next door. But instead of calling her a "fat cow" or a "flat-butt freak," try discussing what she's done to deserve your disapproval, which probably has nothing to do with her body (unless she farted on you). You'll find that when you stop being extremely critical of others, you'll feel better about yourself, too. This is definitely important in your journey to stop body bashing!

"Fat" Substitutions

While you're working on your eating and exercise habits, why not stop the negative body talk, too? Here are some positive, lighthearted alternatives to the "f-word" to help you see yourself (and others) as more than just a jeans size:

Bodacious
Zaftig (means pleasingly plump)
Statuesque
Phat (Pretty Hot and Tempting)
Curvaceous
Full-bodied
Generous
Bootylicious
Juicy

OR SCRAP ALL THIS AND CALL YOURSELF—AND OTHERS

BEAUTIFUL!

Remember this: Just as you don't like the negatives that come with being called "fat," smaller people don't like to be called "bones," "twig," "stick," or other words that can be perceived negatively. Switch out those unkind words for "slim," "slender," or "lean."

Have some favorites that you don't see here? Visit www.nancyredd.com and share!

You LOVE Your Body When You...
STOP FOCUSING ON WEIGHT

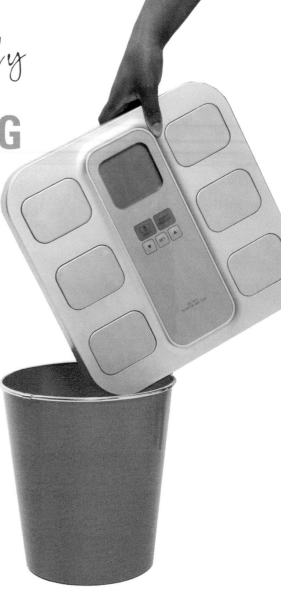

Those tiny little numbers above our toes hold incredible power over our heads! While we're taught to think that our weight is a measure of how much fat and muscle is on our bodies, a large chunk of body weight comes from bones, and amazingly, over half of your body's weight is water. That means that when your weight changes from day to night, it's not because you've gained three pounds in eight hours. It has to do with your hydration levels. Whether you have been sweating it out when you exercise, retaining more of it when you're on your period or after eating something very salty, or dehydrated from not drinking enough of it, your water weight fluctuates an insane amount—up to ten pounds—but this number has very little to do with your fitness and health levels or your long-term clothing size. Add this tidbit of information to the fact that your bones might be a bit bigger than the average girl's, and it's easy to see why it's a good idea to start using other measurements of health that you'll learn about on page 42!

STEP OFF THE SCALE

I HATE SCALES! In *Body Drama* I wrote about kicking my stressful scale-hopping habit. For many of us, myself included, it's not healthy or positive to be jumping on and off the scale all the time, whether once a week, once a day, or once every few hours (as some of us do when struggling with our weight)! Apparently, I'm not alone in my admitted abuse of the scale: More than one in every three teen girls admits to stepping on the scale frequently. Sadly, scale-obsessed girls are more likely to resort to dangerous weight-loss habits such as smoking, taking diet pills, abusing laxatives, skipping meals, and vomiting. And even more maddening, frequent scale use is linked to weight *gain*. One research study weighed teen girls starting in middle school, and five years later, those who said they weighed themselves most often were more than fourteen pounds heavier than those who hardly ever scale-hopped!

So stash your scale for several weeks and see how much better you feel when you wait as long as possible between weigh-ins, especially when you find better ways to measure your health and see that your fitness efforts are paying off!

"Baby Fat"

f.y.i.

Girls often feel "fat" during their tween and teen years because we **do** put on more body fat during that time than boys do—and it's not because we're eating more candy and choco-late! Extra body fat is needed to make us capable of eventually having babies, so don't stress if you feel "rounder" or "fleshier" than usual, because as you grow taller and more womanly, your "baby fat" will likely shift. Don't try to diet it off! Your body needs it. Ironically, to look younger, many women surgically inject fat back **into** parts of their bodies, such as their faces or rears! If it's any consolation, boys at this age often feel wimpy and weak because their muscles don't start developing until they're into their late teens.

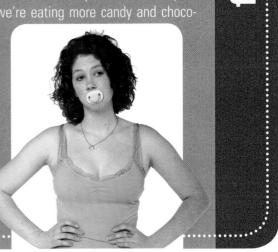

USE BETTER HEALTH MEASUREMENTS

Instead of fretting about the numbers on your scale, focus instead on these alternative health measures:

✿ **Clothing Fit.** Before you start seeing the scale move, you'll usually see a shift in how your jeans fit around your behind and waist. Frequently trying on an old pair of pants or a dress that is one size too small and coming closer and closer to closing that zipper is much more fun than stepping on the stupid scale!

✿ **Measurements.** My favorite way to make sure that I'm making progress is by using my tape measure! In a good week of strength training (see page 98 for more on this), I might not lose weight, but I can see that my leg lifts paid off, firming up my thighs by a quarter-inch, which, combined with the almost-inches lost from other places on my body, adds up to an impressive number. And it's fascinating to see where we tone up—everywhere from our ankles to our wrists and necks— even the jawline can shrink as we get into better shape. Check out page 44 for a fun chart to use in keeping up with your measurements and minimizing the time spent on a scale!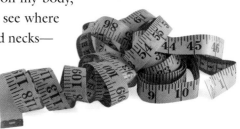

✿ **Waist-to-Hip Ratio.** This calculation isn't perfect, but it's a better measure of health than the Body Mass Index (BMI). The reason is that not all body fat is the same. Having enough body fat is very important, and a little extra padding in various places isn't necessarily a bad thing, but belly fat has the ability to release substances into the blood that can interfere with the body's ability to control blood sugar. This can cause health complications. The waist-to-hip ratio tells you if you have too much belly fat. To find your ratio, divide your waist measurement by your hip measurement. For example, a 29-inch waist and a 39-inch hip gives a waist-to-hip ratio of 29/39 = 0.78). A healthy range for women is between 0.6 and 0.8.

✿ **Strength.** Seeing that first bump of a bicep after a week or two of working out is a really good feeling! So is finding that you can sail through twenty sit-ups when ten used to be a struggle! While clothing fit and inches are great superficial ways to see how well you're progressing toward your goals, becoming stronger is especially good for your soul. Keep track of how much your strength increases by noticing how much easier the exercises on page 119 become, and how many more repetitions you can do before becoming exhausted. Soon you'll be strong enough to smash your scale!

✩ Physical Well-being. Body jiggles and wiggles might never disappear completely, but you'll notice other types of physical improvements when you eat right and exercise! When you move and feed your body properly, you sleep better, have more energy, and won't always need caffeine or a nap to get through the day. Once you know how good it feels to feel good, you'll realize that all your efforts are well worth it!

✩ Emotional Health. Exercising and eating better improves your mood, making it easy to body bash less and love life more. Exercise is good medicine for "the blues," and good food keeps your brain humming along at peak efficiency. The better you feel, the clearer your head will be, and the more you'll realize that a healthy lifestyle is about more than weight loss. The scale is only one way—and perhaps the least important way—to gauge the progress you're making toward good health!

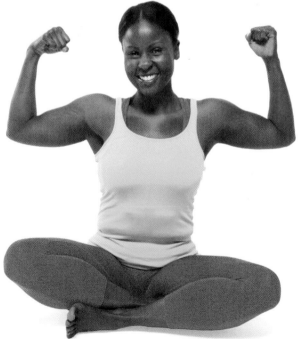

HOW TO: Take Your Measurements

When you're ready to start measuring your body, for the best results make sure that you're wearing nothing but a swimsuit or bra and underwear. Place your feet flat on the ground while keeping your body relaxed and your eyes facing forward. Pull the measuring tape snugly but not tightly, and measure your different body parts at the following locations:

Neck – Around your Adam's apple (the hard spot in the front of your neck).

High Bust – Directly underneath your armpits, above your breasts.

Bust – Fullest part of your bustline.

Waist – Smallest part of your torso.

Belly – Directly over your bellybutton.

Upper Arm – Widest part of your upper arm.

Forearm – Widest part of your forearm.

Wrist – Directly on the wristbone.

Hips – Widest part of your hips.

Upper Thigh – Widest part of your thigh.

Calf - Widest part of your calf.

Ankle – Directly over the anklebone.

NOTE: If you have a friend or a family member that you trust, ask them to measure you for more accurate results. Record your progress on this chart!

Measurements Chart

	WEEK 1	WEEK 2	WEEK 3	WEEK 4	WEEK 5	WEEK 6
NECK						
HIGH BUST						
BUST						
WAIST						
BELLY						
UPPER ARM						
FOREARM						
WRIST						
HIPS						
UPPER THIGH						
CALF						
ANKLE						

Visit www.nancyredd.com for a printable copy of this chart!

You LOVE Your Body When You...
ACCEPT YOUR SHAPE

Here's where body image gets very tricky. We've been brainwashed to believe that the thinner we are, the more attractive we are. We've also been taught to think that thinner means healthier. In a looks lineup, most of us would pick the thinner girl over the thicker one as healthier, but this isn't necessarily true!

(Each of us is born with a certain build.) Just as forces you can't control determine how short or tall you will grow, the genes you inherited from your ancestors have a lot to do with your body shape—whether you are naturally slim in the middle, wide in the hips, heavy in the legs, or small in the chest. Every body shape is beautiful, and any body shape can be healthy. It is also possible for any body shape to be unhealthy, too! No one body type is better, although across a large number of people, some health trends show up. For example, small, petite girls are more likely to develop brittle bones when they get older, and oval-shaped girls face a greater risk of heart disease.

Some girls are naturally thin, but they aren't always physically fit. Cholesterol problems, weak muscles, frequent illnesses, and fatigue can plague slim people, too, especially if they aren't exercising or eating right. No one, no matter their body shape, can get away with unhealthy habits! Even if it looks like a person has no health problems from their outside, there are no guarantees about their insides. Whatever health risks a certain body type faces, it's possible to reduce these risks by eating right and exercising. What *isn't* possible is for people of any shape or size to be healthy without feeding their bodies well and moving their bodies enough!

Contrary to what's been crammed in your head since childhood, it is *absolutely* possible for the size twelve to be healthier than the size two. However, accepting our bodies can be a challenge, especially if we're naturally bigger. Despite Mother Nature's blueprint for our bodies, too many of us resort to harmful habits out of a desire to be thin, whether it's missing meals, binging and purging, or using dangerous diet aids. If this describes you, stop hurting yourself right now and start trying to accept and love your body today!

BTW:
TO BMI OR NOT TO BMI?

I bet you were expecting me to tell you to use your Body Mass Index— BMI for short—to measure health, right? Not in this book! You have probably already heard about BMI from your doctor or at school, but I left this measurement out because although BMI is the most popular way of classifying individuals as overweight or obese, it's more of a shaming tool than an accurate measure of health! Muscles weigh more than fat, and some girls truly have heavier bones, thicker shapes, or stockier builds than others of their age. The result is frequently a BMI number that can erroneously classify a healthy-weight person as overweight or obese.
(See page 147 for a real-life example!)

Success Story: Jen

"Plump, big, fluffy, whatever you want to call it—since I was a child, I was fat. I was singled out all through elementary and middle school. Boys made bets with each other about me, and when one asked me to dance at a school dance, afterwards his friends paid him five dollars. Life at home didn't make things any easier. My parents were both naturally thin people, and they were horrified that I put on weight so easily. They would lock up and hide anything in the house that was even remotely questionable: cookies, chocolate, chips, you name it. That made me feel so ashamed and embarrassed that, when my friends went on a just-stop-eating diet, I did, too. But I wasn't as 'good' at it as they were, and my hunger would cause me to binge later. Over the years, I tried exercising to exhaustion and limiting my food severely. I'd lose and gain and lose again, but overall I saw very little progress pound-wise.

"When I met my now-fiancé, a big guy himself, he would constantly compliment my body. 'What?' I would say. 'You're crazy. I'm not hot, I'm fat.' 'You know,' he'd respond, 'in Yiddish, women like you are called zaftig. It means juicy, and it's a big compliment. It shows that a woman is touchable and soft.'

"After that, I stopped dangerous dieting and started treating my body with respect, nourishing it with good food, and exercising regularly to stay healthy and not to get skinny. It's just that my body pretty much WANTS to look this way, and that's not a bad thing. Now that I've stopped abusing my body, my weight and clothing size have stayed the same for the past five years. Best of all, my self-esteem has shot through the roof! I am VERY, VERY lucky to have a partner who has loved my body, held my hand, and led me into the wonderful world of body love."

LEARN WHAT YOU CAN AND CANNOT CHANGE

First, before embarking on a health-kick, figure out what makes you awesome and unique right now, because no matter how much you lose or gain, those aspects of yourself are here to stay.

Why shouldn't you put so much stock in your size? Many of us truly are born to be bigger, even if we're exercising often and eating healthily. If you are genetically a larger-framed girl, with "meat on your bones" as my mom would say about me, there's a good chance that no matter how much you exercise and how carefully you count calories, you're probably never going to get extremely thin, or if you do, you won't stay there for very long. (I lasted a year as a zero and it was a full-time job. No, really, it was my job! As Miss Virginia I spent hours at the gym and didn't touch candy for an entire year so I could fit into my tiny clothes.) So if you dream of looking like a slender reed, but you are naturally oval-shaped and your bra is a 36C, it's really in your best interest to hold a little mental funeral for the figure you wish you could have (as I had to do with my celebrity worship, page 29) and start believing that health comes in every shape and size, even yours!

fast fact

Your love handles may save your life one day! In 2010, a gunman outside a bar missed his target and instead shot a female bystander. The woman wasn't seriously hurt because the bullet didn't penetrate her fat. She said, "I want to be as big as I can if it's going to stop a bullet!"

Once you start eating better and being active, you might realize that you naturally have a full figure, most of which may not be going anywhere; or you may be surprised to see the inches disappear with your shifts in eating and exercise. Regardless of what you discover, keeping your focus on building a fit, fabulous figure relative to the reality of your bone structure and body shape will benefit you in many ways. Over time, you'll find that getting healthy and staying in great shape become easier as you feel better about yourself, both physically and mentally!

Note that I am NOT saying you should give up your goals of getting into a smaller clothing size, nor am I suggesting that you won't be able to look amazing or enjoy the best health of your life. What I AM saying is that the ideal body type we see in the media might not be the beauty ideal for you. Most of us can be pretty sure that we're never going to end up as six-foot-tall supermodels. But we can all get in the best shape for our bodies, and that's what beauty is for us.

So what should you be working on, and what should you learn to accept? These are very personal questions, but the answers are pretty clear in many cases. Say, for example, that you're from a family where everyone is under five feet tall and over two hundred pounds. Your parents have health issues and take many medications. No one bothers with physical activity at your house, and family time is spent chilling on the couch. Food is usually fried or from fast-food restaurants. Yours might not be the typical TV-sitcom family, but you are far from alone!

(Health starts at home, since you not only get your genes from your family, but also your habits.) You can't change your genes, but you can change your habits. Instead of feeling sorry for yourself because heredity might be keeping you in size twenty-two-short jeans, realize that you have an opportunity to change your current lifestyle for the better. Granted, you'll never shop for a size two-long, but once you've squashed that silly and senseless dream, you can start working toward a healthy lifestyle (As you start exercising and feeling better, you will feel your stress levels decrease and your happiness levels increase, and you can swap your size twenty-two for an eighteen, or even a fourteen someday. Even if your size and shape are more in the average range, the concept stays the same. Setting realistic goals and working to attain them can be fun, whether you are aiming for a size eight or a size eighteen. Impossible goals are doomed to go down in flames along with your self-esteem!

While you can't change your basic body type, you can begin to believe that your appearance doesn't have to determine whether you will find love and have a great life. What will keep you from these things, however, is an unhealthy, unhappy lifestyle. Eating nothing except junk and moping around all day are surefire ways to ruin your health and deny yourself happiness. So snap out of your pity party, accept your shape, and make the choice to live your life to its healthiest and its fullest!

WORK WITH WHAT YOU HAVE

Once you stop body bashing and accept your unique shape, the only beauty ideal for you is YOU—at your best! Remember that accepting and appreciating your body as-is doesn't mean giving up. It means that, instead of stressing about what you can't change, you start making the changes that are right for you. After you cut out the crushing comparisons that got you nowhere fast, you can start to work with what you have, not with what you wish you had! You can begin to figure out what looks good on your shape.

You might have a peachy personality, but your body may be all pear! While weight can and will fluctuate, for the most part your body shape will stay the same; a pancake butt will probably stay flat no matter how much weight you gain, and those broad shoulders aren't budging no matter what diet you pursue. Accepting your body and working with what you have means having an eye for what looks good on you, not necessarily limiting yourself to the season's latest style. Some trends don't flatter certain body types; they can look terrible even on supermodels! Something from last season that looks sensational on you will take you a lot further than a trendy top that's too tight.

There are five basic body types, and they are named for items that look like the shape they represent: oval, triangle, inverted triangle, rectangle, and "X." Learning which one most resembles your body and using your type to figure out what flatters your figure can go a long way toward helping you to look your best.

BTW: DIETS ARE OLD NEWS

The word **diet** comes from the Greek word **diaeta**, which means "way of living," and diet books have a history that goes back some 2,500 years. The ancient Greeks were obsessed with health manuals and exercise handbooks penned by an array of experts and doctors, all of whom offered contradictory advice. Sound familiar?

Body Acceptance vs. Body Avoidance

Some people use the phrase "body acceptance" in the proper way, meaning that you accept what you cannot change about your body and adjust your beauty ideals to look more like yourself. But sometimes we also use "body acceptance" to avoid dealing with the difficulty of discussing and working on our bodies. When you're depressed, scared, angry, or just in a bad place, it's easy to say that you've simply "accepted" your body "as-is" when what you really mean is that you're down in the dumps and you don't know how to do anything about your concerns! Body acceptance does NOT mean strapping yourself to the sofa, putting your favorite pizza place on speed dial, wearing nothing but an oversize T-shirt, shutting yourself off from fun activities such as going to the beach or school dances, and pretending that you're happy and fine. Sound extreme? Think about it. When was the last time you worked up a sweat that wasn't temperature related? Ate a vegetable without gravy, butter, or cheese? Gave your back and legs a good, groan-worthy stretch? Let's face the facts. Many of us live lazy lives. Our laziness has nothing to do with our bodies and everything to do with our minds. When we decide to love ourselves and our bodies, we start to value how lucky we are. We look for ways to make the most of life, and we look forward to an exciting future of keeping our bodies and our brains nourished and nurtured. On the other hand, when you don't respect your body and when you feel bad about yourself, what motivation do you have to put down that third piece of pizza? There's nothing else to get excited about!

I'm not saying that you need to lose weight to look and feel great, but you do need to work on your health. No young woman, large or small, should ever live in fear of waking up to find herself fused to her computer chair weighing five hundred pounds! No one needs or wants inactivity, an unhealthy diet, and a distressed mind. So what are you waiting for? If you don't already, begin to believe that you deserve to feel good and take care of yourself, no matter what your size!

BODY TYPES

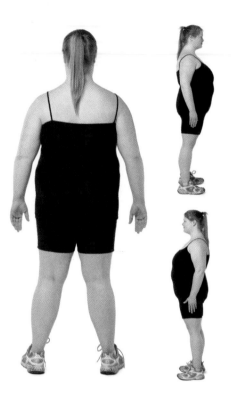

The Oval - O

Is your waist wider than your shoulders and hips? Do you mostly gain weight around your middle and/or your chest? Ovals look oh-so-lovely in empire-waist dresses, straight-leg pants and jeans, sleeveless tops, shorter skirts, and tops that don't need to be tucked in.

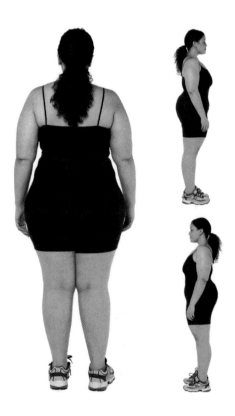

The Triangle - ▲

Are your hips wider than your shoulders? Do you usually gain weight in your bottom and hips? Triangles look tantalizing in flared skirts, boot-legged pants and jeans, empire-waist dresses, and tops and jackets that come to the hipbone (which is about the same level as where your pubic hair begins).

The Inverted Triangle - ▼

Are your shoulders wider than your hips? Are you frequently called "broad-shouldered" or "athletic-looking"? Inverted triangles look incredible in "V" necklines, full skirts, pants and jeans with pockets, and tunic tops.

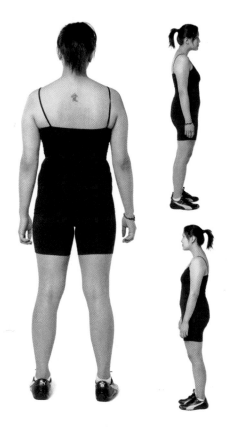

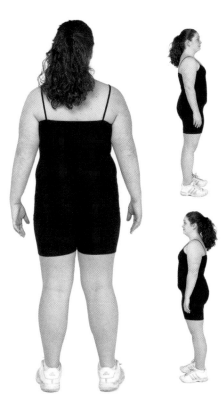

The Rectangle - ▮

Are you straight up and down, without a defined waist? When you gain weight, does it settle all over? Rectangles look ravishing in sheath dresses, striped or patterned tops with a solid-colored bottom, flared skirts, and jackets that come to the hipbone.

The "X" - X

Are your shoulders and hips about the same width? Is your waist clearly defined? Do you gain weight all over and not in one specific area? X-shaped girls look great in tucked-in shirts, fitted clothing, straight skirts, and belted pants and jeans.

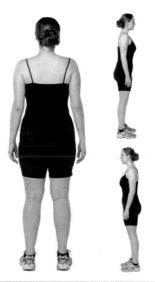

Stop Rejecting Compliments!

If your BFF says to you, "Wow, you look nice today!" which is the correct response?

a. "OMG, I look **soooo** bad!" (even though you spent hours getting dressed)

b. A dirty look because you're sure she's being sarcastic.

c. "I'm trying, but I couldn't get my hair right, and did you see this stain?"

d. "Thanks!"

You know that D is the **right** choice, but sometimes what comes out of your mouth may be your insecurity speaking for you. We tend to think it's totally normal to talk dirt about ourselves (and one another), but when it comes to playing nice we're so used to putting ourselves down that we don't know how to get in the game! As you start to improve yourself, people are going to notice, and that's a good thing. You might feel self-conscious or embarrassed, but you don't have to put yourself down or brush off someone's attempt to be nice to you. Even if you suspect sarcasm, when someone says something complimentary, don't let your mind start racing to find ways to downplay it. Just accept it!

The next time someone notices your good looks, try a simple "thank you." Your thanks say that you appreciate the compliment, at the same time sending a signal to your brain to start believing in yourself. And get used to compliments! The better you take care of yourself, the more positive comments you'll hear!

HOW TO Carry Yourself Well!

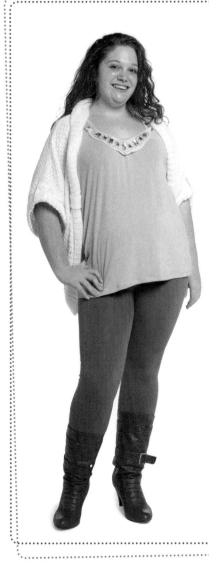

Whether you're into the latest trends or not, confidence is always in season. Some of us seem to have been born confident, but for most of us, confidence requires work for our entire lives. It's worth the effort! Carrying yourself with confidence improves your looks more than an entirely new wardrobe, so:

☆ Practice good posture (stop slouching).

☆ Make eye contact (especially with your crush).

☆ Be the first to say hello and ask people about their day.

☆ When someone compliments you, don't reject the kind words. Simply say, "Thanks!"

☆ Keep your hands by your side. Don't cross them as if you have something to hide.

☆ SMILE!

These steps ensure that, even if you're a little worried about how you look, you won't give off an insecure vibe. Try out these tips and see how other people react!

Medical Health Tests

Curious to find out more about your health from the inside out? Schedule the following tests with your doctor as soon as possible, especially if you're starting to change your lifestyle:

✫ **Blood Pressure.** You know that arm-cuff thingie that you see in pharmacies? Take advantage of it the next time you spy one, or ask your doctor to explain your numbers when you have a checkup. Blood pressure is a measure of the health of your circulatory system (blood, heart, arteries, and veins). A healthy blood pressure range is between 90/60 and 120/70.

✫ **Cholesterol.** One in five teens has a cholesterol problem, whether it's not enough of the good kind (HDL) or too much of the bad kind (LDL). Some also have higher levels of another kind of fat in the blood, called triglycerides. With a quick blood test (don't let a fear of needles stop you), your doctor can find out if you're in that 20 percent. The problem with bad cholesterol is that it clogs up your arteries and leads to heart disease. Cholesterol issues aren't always linked to poor diet and exercise, so it's important to get checked out if you're wondering about your health, regardless of your fitness and food habits. (Read more on cholesterol on page 223.) When you get your results back, see if they're in the healthy range (as measured in milligrams per deciliter of blood). For adults those levels are LDL below 100, HDL above 60, and triglycerides below 150. Ask your doctor what's right for your age.

✫ **Blood Glucose Levels.** This test will show you how well your body is handling glucose, the body's main source of energy. If your blood glucose rises too high, this can cause damage to your eyes, kidneys, nerves, and blood vessels. A level that is too low is not desirable either. It can cause nervousness, sweating, intense hunger, and weakness. Your doctor can measure your blood glucose in several different ways. A healthy measurement after you have fasted for eight hours or more should be somewhere between 70 and 100 (milligrams per deciliter).

fast fact

Knowing your body shape can help your health as well as your clothes shopping. Statistically, the oval body shape (also known as the apple) is associated with a greater risk of heart disease, breast cancer, and diabetes because of the extra belly fat. On the other hand, triangle (pear)- shaped women are more prone to osteoporosis (brittle bones), varicose veins, and image issues such as eating disorders and poor self-esteem.

When Medical Concerns Cause Weight Gain

Have you ever wanted to scream, "I HAVE A MEDICAL ISSUE, MORON" at someone who makes a crass comment, suggesting that laziness is to blame for your increasing size? It can be devastating to find out that there's no healthy way to shed extra weight that comes from certain medical circumstances. "Calories in" might NOT mean "calories out" for your body as it does for most people. Common issues that cause weight gain or the inability to slim down include the following:

✩ **Certain medications.** As many as fifty different prescription drugs, including those used to treat depression, epilepsy, headaches, diabetes, and high blood pressure can all cause weight gain. Some steroids (the legal kind prescribed by a doctor), hormones, and birth control pills can add pounds, too. But weight gain is no reason to stop taking a prescribed medication. A few extra pounds may be a reasonable trade-off when major health issues are involved!

✩ **Tumors and abnormal hormones.** This category includes, but isn't limited to, Cushing syndrome, in which a tumor grows in the pituitary gland; blood sugar imbalances that cause insulin production to go crazy; hypothyroidism (an underactive thyroid gland), which affects the body's growth and ability to properly process food energy; and polycystic ovary syndrome (a.k.a PCOS) that causes the body to create too much male hormone, often causing weight gain.

✩ **Inactivity due to a (visible or invisible) physical disability.** While there are ways to work around limitations to get some exercise, people with disabilities can have a tough time trimming down.

If you're dealing with a disease or disorder, getting your body healthy trumps slimming down. You may have a hard time accepting that your body may not look exactly the way you want it to, at least not for now. But remember, weight loss isn't the only reason to feed your body healthy foods and, if your doctor approves, to move your body often. Good food and exercise improve your mood and the way your body feels. They can have a positive effect on your medical condition, too. But whether you think you have something wrong or not, you MUST see your doctor before changing your exercise routine or eating habits. And NEVER stop taking your medicines or following doctor's orders just because of weight gain.

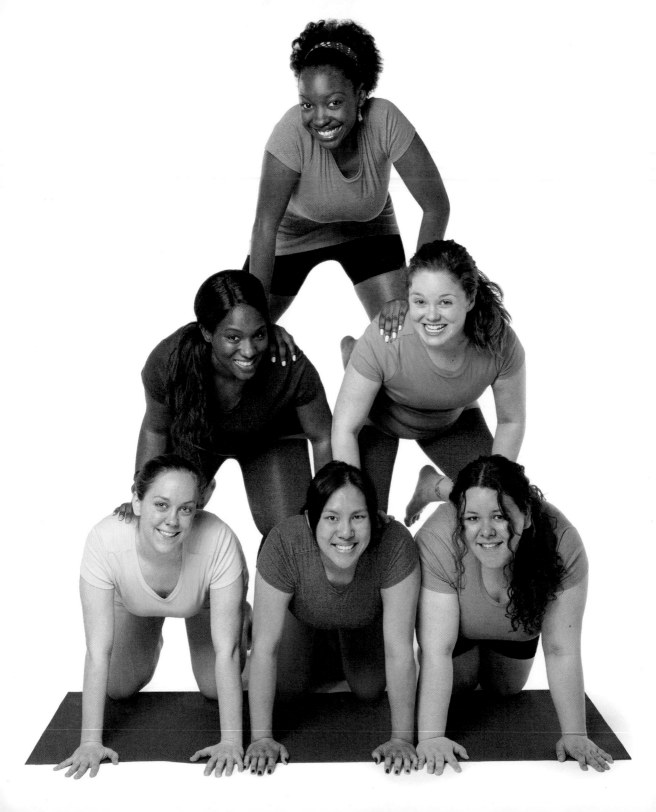

Love Your Body
DRAMAS

I can't enjoy my life until my body is better.

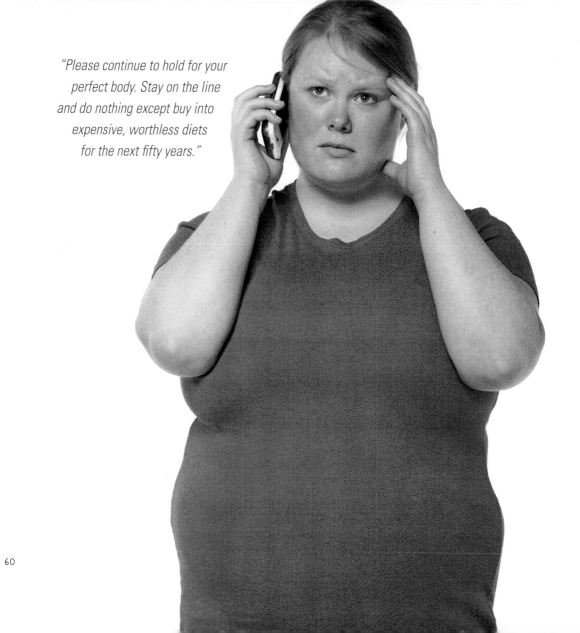

"Please continue to hold for your perfect body. Stay on the line and do nothing except buy into expensive, worthless diets for the next fifty years."

WHAT'S GOING ON?

I'm sure no one would want to date me because of my body, so why flirt?

I won't be chosen for the team because of my weight, so why bother trying?

I hate the way I look in my swimsuit, so why go to the beach?

I can't fit into what everyone else is wearing, so what's the point of trying to look cute?

Do you use the size of your behind to back out of having a good time? You're not alone! The diet industry has fooled many of us into believing that life isn't worth living until we have the body of a beauty ideal, or at least a better body than the one we have now. That idea is both unfair and untrue!

You may think that everything will be wonderful once you reach your body goals, but realistically you may need months or years to get there. You can't put life on hold until then! You can't pause the party until you reach perfection because you'll be wasting tons of time that you'll never get back, leaving blank spaces in your life history that you could be filling with memories, experiences, accomplishments, and most important, *fun*. There is no rewind or erase button built into your life, so don't waste some of the most exciting years of your life on frustration and failed diets!

It's easy to blame your body for ruining your life. Going after dreams and goals is challenging, and you may feel tempted to use a less-than-perfect body as an excuse to never start. We hide behind our size as a way to avoid the difficulties that come with showing people how smart, funny, interesting, and worthy we really are. Hiding seems easier, but it makes things harder in the long run.

HOW DO I DEAL?

There is NOTHING wrong with wanting to improve yourself, and this book is full of healthy ways to help you do just that, but it's a terrible idea to wait until the finish line to live your life to the fullest. There's so much amazing stuff in store along the way, so:

✪ **Stop scapegoating.** The first step is small, but has a big impact: Stop using your body as a scapegoat! What's a scapegoat? It's an old term for something you single out to blame instead of facing the real problem. You're scapegoating when you tell yourself and others that you can't enjoy life until your body looks better.

✪ **Start saying YES.** The next time you're faced with a challenging obstacle or a cool opportunity, say yes instead of turning away! Start small at first. Accept invitations to hang out, dare to bare your bod in a bathing suit instead of putting off the pool, and raise your hand in class when you know the answer. You can work your way up from there.

✪ **Strive to be positive.** When you start taking on new challenges, try to start thinking and talking about your body in better ways, too. Change the way you carry yourself and talk about your body (stop body bashing!), and eventually positive thinking will become second nature!

When you show more respect for your body, you'll probably notice a change in how other people treat you. That's because a big part of the way others see you comes from the messages you send about what you deserve. Still, when you put yourself out there and start living large, you might find your voyage is not always smooth sailing, regardless of your size. No one likes being rejected, but no matter what you do, you might not make the team, make friends with the cool kids, or find love with that special someone. *But that's not your body's fault!* That's life, and EVERYONE, regardless of size, gets rejected once in a while. You will end up better off if you move on and keep trying for the things you want in life! You will eventually achieve your goals, and you'll be proud that you didn't let your body keep you from getting to where you wanted to go.

Low Self-Esteem and Body Image

Low self-esteem can put an emotional load on our already stressed shoulders that we don't need, especially when we're working on our health. Do you:

- often think, when you hear people laugh, that they must be laughing about you?

- hate answering your phone or reading your texts or e-mails because you're afraid someone is going to be rude?

- dread having to talk in class because you don't want any attention to be focused on you?

- have trouble trusting others or feel quick to cut-off relationships for fear that someone will hurt you or cut you off first?

- constantly tell yourself how stupid, ugly, unlovable, weird, or otherwise awful you are?

- see a less-than-bright future ahead for yourself?

If you answered yes to any of those questions, you may be struggling with poor self-esteem. Maybe these symptoms crept up from the body blues, but they come from a place in your mind that weight loss alone won't change. Such feelings are common among young women, but they aren't healthy. If your self-esteem is low, talk with a trusted adult, such as your guidance counselor, school nurse, parent, guardian, or doctor. Share your feelings. Don't keep them bottled up inside. If you do, they'll only get worse.

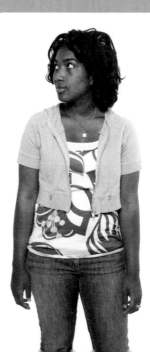

I CONFESS: I DIDN'T WAIT FOR WEIGHT LOSS!

One of the accomplishments I'm most known for is winning the swimsuit competition at the Miss America Pageant, but that was one of the only times in my life when I've been what you could call thin. I'm naturally a "bootylicious" girl and, for me, being smaller than a size six or eight is a full-time job that I have no interest in applying for again anytime soon. Of all the years in my life, I've been "thin" for fewer than four. But my size never stopped me from achieving my goals. Here are some of the awesome achievements I would have missed if I had waited for weight loss:

- ✩ Captain of my cheerleading squad (size ten-twelve)

- ✩ School president (size ten-twelve)

- ✩ Accepted into Harvard University (size twelve)

- ✩ Senior prom (size twelve)

- ✩ Won $250K on **Who Wants to Be a Millionaire?** (size twelve)

- ✩ And many more!

If I had twiddled my thumbs in anticipation of those few months when I'd get down to a size zero, I wouldn't have accomplished anything along the way. Even at the Miss Virginia competition, many beautiful women looked more like the media's beauty ideal than I did, but my accomplishments and the person I became at my "regular" weight enabled me to win the title! Remember this as you go after the life you want to live: Always strive for success regardless of your size!

I am TIRED of people calling me fat!

WHAT'S GOING ON?

Sticks and stones may break my bones,
but words can never hurt me.

"Did she just say what I think she said?!"

(Yeah, right. Whoever wrote that old saying had never been ragged on.)

Let's face the truth: Words hurt. I'm always amazed by how insensitive some people can be when commenting on size and shape. I've had stuff said to me that tore me up inside more than a blow to the stomach ever could . . . BY PEOPLE WHO LOVE ME! Passive comments, friendly teasing, or malicious bullying can make you feel bad, as can those well-meaning friends and family members who call you "fat" because they're trying to "help motivate you" to lose the weight. If you're like me, those comments make you feel annoyed, angry, or tearful. Teasing and bashing hurt enough when the words aren't true (You're so stupid you once returned donuts because they had holes in them!), but they hurt even more when they contain a grain of truth, especially about weight. ("You're as wide as flat-screen TV!" My flat screen measures only fifteen inches across, so, yes, I AM wider than a flat-screen TV.)

People call you fat for two main reasons:

Reason #1: They want to feel superior. While you may be the target, the nasty comment isn't about you. Bullies, jerks, and insecure friends often think that the worse they can make others feel, the better they'll look. They are wrong! Busy, happy, confident people do not make fun of others. They have better things to do. Unfortunately, our world (especially in middle and high school) is full of unhappy, insecure individuals who choose to mask their problems by making fun of other people, including you and me! So when you're trying your best to ignore soul-crushing comments, remember where they're coming from.

fast fact

Not surprising: 60 percent of middle school bullies have been convicted of a crime by age twenty-four.

Reason #2: They want to help. Moms, dads, mentors, and other well-meaning people who care about you fall into this category. They believe that your health and/or social life are in danger, and they consider their rude remarks "tough love" or "keepin' it real." Ironically, their shaming comments don't motivate! Even if you want to slim down some, you may find yourself rebelling against the criticism. In that case, no one wins.

HOW DO I DEAL?

It would be easy for me to say, "Ignore them, girlfriend. The only voice that matters is in your mind!" But I know that dealing with negative comments is more complicated than that. So try to hang tight with these tactics:

✿ Translate. Even if you do have a lot of jiggle in your wiggle, a bully who says, "You're FAT!" is really saying, "I want my words to be as painful as possible, and your body is the most obvious thing I can use to bring you down, so I hope I can make you feel bad with what I say." Don't let your critic succeed. When those who love you call you fat, they're saying, "The world is harder for heavy people and I read a magazine article that said heavy people have more health problems and I do not want that for you so I'm going to make you face the truth to force you to start shaping up so that your life can be great." Those messages may be sent with good intentions, but the emotional consequences can be catastrophic.

When you understand what people are trying to say—whether good or bad—you can ignore what doesn't matter and think about what does—knowing that YOU can and will decide what to do about your body.

✿ Stay calm. Whether you ignore the comment or simply walk away, try to stay cool and collected. That means no yelling back and no crying, no matter how upset you may be! Confrontation can cause fat-talk to worsen, and you probably can't get your point across anyway. Being rude right back might escalate the situation to some kind of fight, which you don't want. The less affected you seem, the more fat-talkers are likely to move on to other subjects.

✿ Keep your focus. While perfecting your poker face on the outside, you may have to work equally hard to control how you feel inside. Realize that even a label that's true—for example, "four-eyes" if you wear glasses or "big butt" if your rear is large—doesn't have to hurt. Those aspects of yourself aren't bad. They're just parts of you! Don't let mere words cause you to start a crazy diet, dabble in destructive behaviors, or give up on your goals. Striving for success is the best way to win, as you'll prove to the haters and the taunters how powerless they are over you.

✿ Tell someone. Don't accept bullying in silence. Tell someone that you're not being treated well, even if you don't want to get the basher in trouble. Confiding in someone you trust, such as a close friend, family member, teacher, guidance counselor, or minister, is better for you than keeping your emotions bottled up. You don't have to confront or call out the teaser, but you don't have to ignore the way the taunts tear you up either. Internalizing negative comments can damage your self-esteem. You'll deal better if you get support from someone close to you who will say, "That (nasty comment) is totally not true!"

belly laughs

Doc says to girl, "I'm not liking the way your X-rays look. Your liver and heart both are enlarged and don't look healthy." Girl replies, "Can't you just airbrush them so that they're smaller?"

Really Bad Bullying

Bullies often notice when their target is trying to improve, so they ramp up their wretched behavior and take things far past teasing. Be prepared for that possibility, and don't let fear stop you from improving your life. Push forward with your personal goals, put things in perspective, and keep trusted adults in the loop. If your friends are bullying you, try to find new groups of people to hang with—if not in school then in your community—so you have a separate bunch of friends who don't know the bashers and can't be influenced by them. If bashing becomes physical or turns into extremely painful verbal abuse (attacking your character or ethnicity), you HAVE to report the abuser to your school counselor or principal before the situation takes a turn for the worse. You might not think that the adults at your school care, but they do. They know that bullying can prompt some young people to think about suicide, and they want to keep their students alive and well. Present your case clearly and truthfully. You WILL be heard!

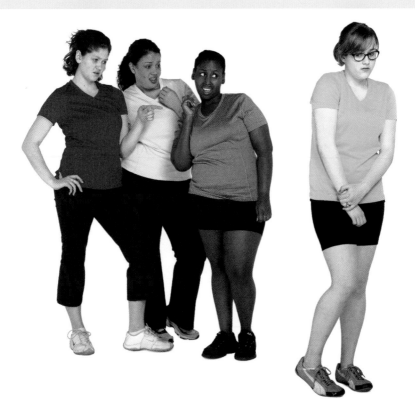

Strange Sizing

Are you peeved when you find that a size ten is too small when you're usually a perfect eight? Don't worry. We all have that experience! Each clothing designer chooses his or her own standard for sizing. Some designers cut their clothing small, while others leave room to spare. Check out Allie in the pictures below as she tries on three pairs of the same-sized pants from different companies. Some pants are like parachutes; others she can't even zip! Just goes to show: Size isn't everything. Find the flattering outfit that fits your body and not the clothing size you wish you wore!

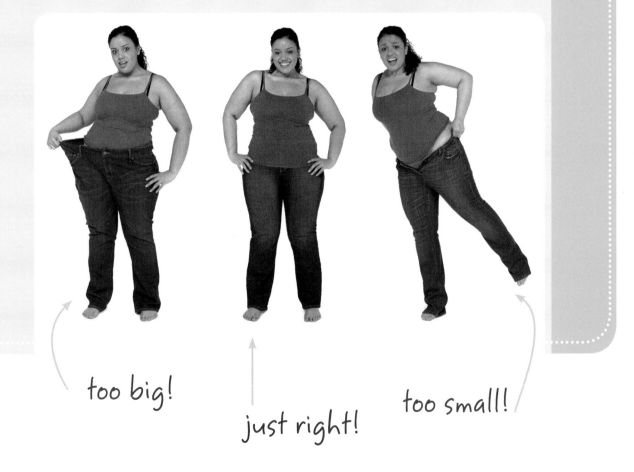

too big!

just right!

too small!

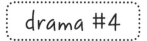

I just want to have
weight-loss surgery
and be done with it!

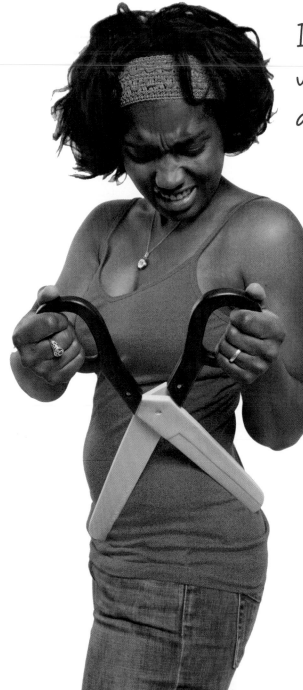

WHAT'S GOING ON?

Sorry to burst your bubble, but you WON'T be done with worrying about your weight after surgery, and here's the thing: You might be DONE forever! Although the number of weight loss operations performed on teenagers has recently tripled, surgery still kills, even the so-called simple procedures used to treat obesity. If you think weight-loss surgery is 100 percent safe, think again. The risks are no small potatoes! One out of every 100 people who have weight-loss surgery dies during or right after the operation and another five die within five years. Even for large numbers of those who survive, the procedure causes severe and permanent complications! Nearly half, for example, end up iron deficient, and as many as a third develop painful gallstones within six months after the surgery. Such risks make weight-loss surgery an option only as a last resort.

"But this IS a last resort," you might be thinking. Before saying that out loud, are you SURE? Prior to rushing off to the surgeon's office, you have to really look at weight-loss surgery for what it is: a major operation causing permanent, inconvenient, and sometimes painful changes to your body that you will have to deal with for the rest of your life. Don't get me wrong, there truly are some teens for whom weight-loss surgery is the right choice . . . and then, more than likely . . . there's you. If you believe surgery is a shortcut that will force you into the eating habits you've failed to develop on our own, you're off track! Though you might see it talked about on television all of the time, weight-loss surgery is rarely for teens because of potential health complications. Some develop brittle bones and other health problems in their late teens and early twenties because of their lack of nutrition after the surgery, even with careful monitoring and medication.

Even worse, the surgery is no guarantee of weight loss. Nearly one in every five patients fail to lose even half the weight they were hoping to. And even those who do face a lifetime of dietary restrictions. One popular weight-loss surgery shrinks your stomach to the size of a thumb (down from a fist), so that if you eat more than a few ounces at a time or eat too quickly, you instantly feel the urge to throw up. Now that will teach you portion control fast! Another surgery reroutes food from the stomach around a part of the small intestine, meaning the body absorbs far fewer nutrients and calories. Sounds good, right? Maybe, but nearly 70 percent of patients experience long-term vomiting as a result of that surgery, not to mention gas, abdominal pains, nausea, weakness, sweating, diarrhea, fainting, and more. They also face severe restrictions on what they can eat. Anything containing fat or sugar is hard to digest, and many doctors recommend avoiding nuts and seeds, popcorn, dried fruits, some cereals, stringy or fibrous vegetables, tough meats, and bread. Many kids who undergo weight-loss surgery are never, ever allowed to drink soda, either, whether it's sugar-free or not, because the carbonation can cause intense stomach pain. That doesn't leave much to enjoy, does it? Whether you let the surgeons cut you open or not, you'll eventually need to learn how to eat right and exercise, it's just that with the surgery you'll be a lot more restricted!

If you're in constant fear of pain or pooping your pants, of course it's easier to eat only healthy foods and lose weight! But think about what you have done: YOU HAVE PAID SOMEONE TO CHANGE YOUR BODY FOREVER SO YOU CAN LIVE IN CONSTANT FEAR OF THROWING UP OR POOPING YOUR PANTS! Can you imagine that fate for even one week? How about forty to sixty years of never being able to have a whole hot dog just because you were impatient as a teen? And then, after all of that, the weight loss might not be permanent. Your stomach may stretch back to its normal size, or your body might adapt to needing fewer calories to survive, making the surgery useless.

HOW DO I DEAL?

We all get impatient and want what we can't have . . . and we want it yesterday! But whether you're considering a tattoo, a nose job, or weight-loss surgery, you should sit with the desire for as long as possible and talk it through with professionals who can help you to make a sensible choice—one that's right for you both now and in the future. Just as a seventy-five-year-old lady would look ridiculous with a gun tattooed on her tush, she might also feel miserable if she couldn't eat a piece of cake at her seventy-fifth[th] birthday party or if she walked with crutches because a calcium deficiency made her hip bones brittle and malformed. So if you're seriously considering weight-loss surgery, try the following steps to determine if you really want (or need) it or if you just want a quick fix:

★ Figure out WHY you're desperate. And yes, if you're considering surgery, you're desperate, and you've probably convinced yourself that your body is the biggest problem in your life. Whenever that level of importance, nay, desperation, is placed on ANYTHING, emotions and anxieties overwhelm common sense. But if you're in good enough shape to have the surgery safely, you may well be in good enough shape to lose weight *without* a stomach staple or an intestinal bypass. Oftentimes, nothing is stopping you except your mind.

★ Pretend you did it—seriously! Play-act how you think your habits would change once you had the surgery. If you think dieting is no fun now, when you have a choice, imagine how it might be when you have no choice. You may decide you don't need the surgery to improve your eating habits. You can play the role on your own—without the expense, the pain, or the risks.

★ Learn about other options. Eating right and exercising are your other options (conveniently presented in this book) for achieving the same goals as with surgery, perhaps a little more slowly, but with long-lasting and healthier results. Before you take weight-loss surgery seriously, your doctor will probably tell you to try to lose weight the "old-fashioned" way for at least six months. Be fair to your body and give yourself a good shot at getting healthy naturally before you have your belly cut open. Don't know how to get healthy without surgery? You're in luck. That's what the rest of this book is about: learning to be conscious of your everyday eating and exercise habits so that you can achieve your goals without surgery.

Dealing with Doctor Drama

f.y.i.

Heavier people are generally thought of as less healthy than thinner people, but the problem isn't just size, it's shame. Larger people may dread going to the doctor for fear of being chastised about their size, so they wait until something is horribly wrong before seeking help. Don't let this be you! If you're starting to get healthy, even if you have a long way to go, see your doctor for a checkup and start taking care of your body from the inside out.

I need to slim down so much I don't know where to begin!

WHAT'S GOING ON?

The truth is, you DO know where to begin: with the same single clothing size that we all do, whether you're trying to shed a single size or six sizes. When you compare your weight or your size with what the charts say is healthy, you may feel scared, frustrated, or defeated. Fight those feelings! Keep in mind that your health and your happiness don't come from numbers. They come from how you choose to live your life. You'll start to feel a sense of control over both the first time you order a grilled chicken sandwich (hold the mayo) instead of the fried chicken tenders, or the first time you walk up the stairs to the second floor instead of taking the elevator. Loving your body is a lifelong marathon, not a quick race around the corner!

belly laughs

Girl says to doc, "OMG, my tum is so big and I'm totally embarrassed about it." Doc asks, "Have you ever tried to diet?" Girl responds, "Yeah, but not a single color I've tried hides it. It still sticks out!"

HOW DO I DEAL?

First, stop thinking about the end result and start thinking about your journey. Getting fit is a fabulous experience! The first time you can run a mile without breaking a sweat . . . the first time you can do fifty crunches without a single cramp . . . those are priceless moments. You deserve to experience the good feelings that come from working out and taking control of your body! So what are you waiting for? Work it, girl! Gear up and get started on learning how to lose weight in smart and healthy ways. Just give yourself a month. What's the worst-case scenario? You lose thirty days, but I bet you lose a lot more than that, and I mean in a good way!

Trying Dangerous Things to Slim Down

When you choose junk over healthy food or opt out of exercise, you probably aren't purposely trying to sabotage your health. Maybe you feel too lazy to prepare a healthy snack or maybe you like the taste of cheese pizza better than you like cabbage. But when you purposely try dangerous things to lose weight, you've got a big problem that starts with your mind and affects your body. If you take diet pills, starve yourself, take laxatives, or exercise to the point of exhaustion, you are choosing to put thinness above your health. Why? Because you see your body as nothing more than the clothing size you so desperately want it to fit into. Dangerous weight-loss behaviors scream "bad body image." They are no way to reach your goals!

First things first. Immediately stop doing anything to your body that you think might be remotely dangerous. Even if you are seeing positive results on the outside, as with everything, it's the inside that counts; you could be harming your future health by weakening your heart, liver, and even your womb. Next, if you're taking diet pills—even over-the-counter "natural" ones—do some research to find out more about the product. Get information about the ingredients that are listed on the label; you might be surprised by some of the scary reports you find! Finally, talk to someone you can trust. If your desire to lose weight has gone so far that you are hurting yourself, you need professional help. And there's nothing wrong with that! We all need some support sometimes (I talk about my time in therapy in *Body Drama*) and diet and exercise abuse are warning signs that it's time to start talking to someone.

Turn to page 184 for information on diet supplements and eating disorders to learn more.

BTW : EATING DISORDERS AREN'T JUST BAD HABITS!

Anorexia and bulimia are more than bad habits that need to be broken; they're disorders that require medical help. You don't have to be thin to be suffering from one of these eating disorders, either. Anorexia is not just excessive thinness; it's about distorted body image and a reluctance, or inability, to eat, and it can also occur in people who are normal weight. Bulimia is the "purging disorder." Most who have it are of normal weight or heavier. These disorders may not always show on the outside, but the pain their victims feel on the inside is intense. See page 184 for more on these and other disorders.

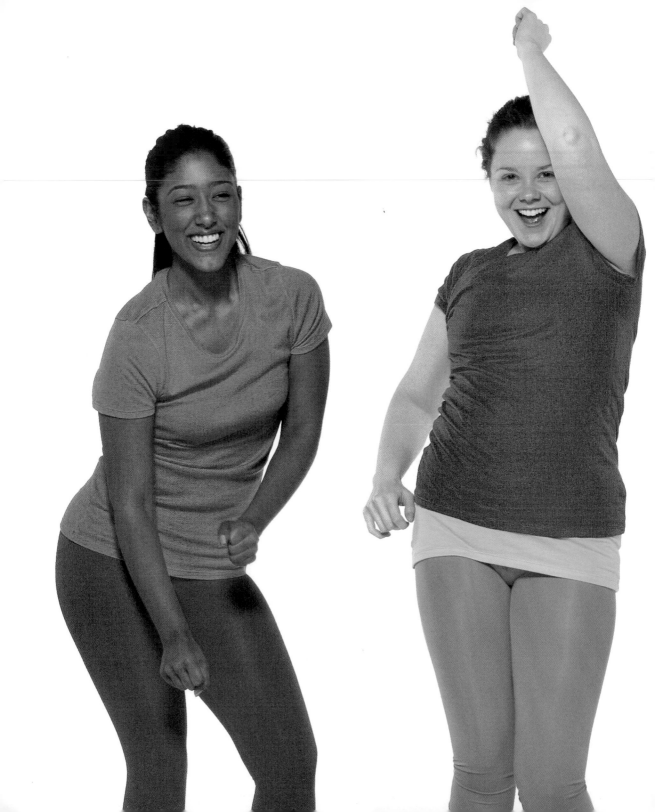

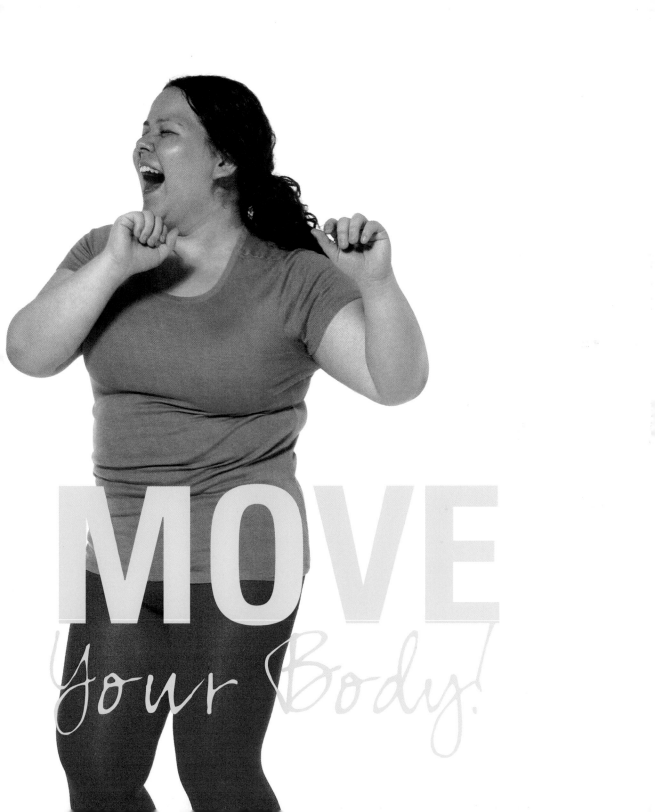

MOVE
Your Body!

"*FOUR MORE REPEATS,*" I yelled, my extra-large gray bike shorts soaked black with sweat. "THREE . . . TWO . . . ONE . . . NOW WALK IT OFF . . . GREAT JOB!" I toweled off to clapping from six or seven adult women who were panting like a pack of animals. As a sixteen-year-old aerobics instructor at a small local gym, I wasn't nervous at all! I knew my routine backward and forward, as I'd been teaching the same class every Monday for a couple of months by now. Most of my moves—and my mixtape—were from my cheerleading squad's routines, which as co-captain, I had helped to make up. I loved every minute of my weekly workout class as well as my hundreds of cheer practice hours—not to mention game nights! Sure, my uniform was one of the largest, but I thought that I looked pretty good in it, and I was in great shape. You should have seen my jumps!

At that time in my life, exercise was so much fun I couldn't get enough of it, but as soon as that mental size-switch flipped in my head during my senior year and I started seeing my body as something that needed to improve, my views on exercise began to change, too. School was almost over and I wasn't on the squad or teaching aerobics anymore, so the workout choices available to me seemed more mind-numbing than the worst of chores. That was

Make moving your body a fun habit, not only to achieve

before televisions were at every workout machine at the gym, so I had to stick it out on the treadmill with my CD player and last month's magazines. At that time, my goal of losing weight before going to college far exceeded my boredom, so I spent all summer at the gym, only to quit cold turkey once I arrived at college. The only thing that got me exercising again was packing the pounds back on! Although I knew the importance of working up a good sweat on a regular basis, my dread of the dreary gym outweighed my interest in weight control. Finally, I discovered a couple of forms of exercise I really enjoyed: yoga, and more recently, triking (yes, triking, see page 139). Sure, there are activities that burn many more calories, but I'm honest with myself: If I don't enjoy an activity, I'll never do it, so doing what I like means I win in both health and happiness!

Now, instead of an unhealthy all-or-nothing exercise routine, most days I can be found triking around outside or doing some sort of yoga. A few times a week I try to tone up my abs, arms, and legs using the exercises starting on page 119. In this chapter, I'll show you some fun ways to exercise that I hope will help you make moving your body a fun habit, not only to achieve short-term shaping-up goals but also for a lifetime!

short-term shaping-up goals but also for a lifetime!

WHAT DOES IT MEAN TO MOVE *My Body?*

We're constantly moving our bodies in order to get through the day, from walking to class to scrubbing ourselves in the shower. But moving your body for health reasons is different from everyday activity, even if your heart rate does go up when you see your crush or if you work up a sweat during a pop quiz!

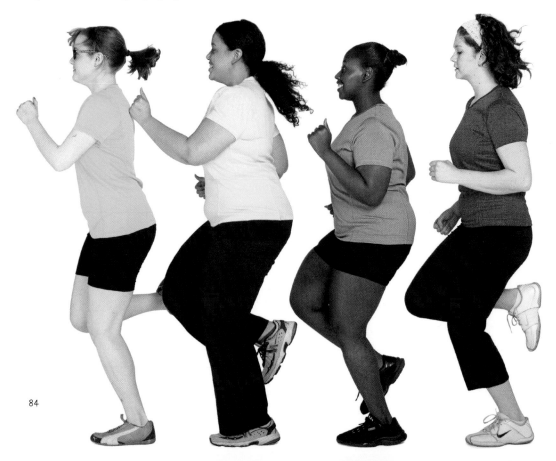

Stretching, strengthening, and sweating help keep your excess body fat levels down and your health and fitness levels up. Think about exercise this way: You trim your split ends to keep your hair healthy, and you wash the dirt off your face to keep it from breaking out, don't you? You need to move your body to keep it healthy, strong, and in shape, too.

We don't always have control over how much we are able to move our bodies, also known as our activity level. Sometimes we fall ill or have physical challenges beyond our control that keep our activity level down (see page 102 for more on this). However, most of us who aren't moving our bodies don't realize how important activity is, not just for our figures but also for our health and well-being! In fact, nearly two out of every three high school students don't get enough exercise! It's really easy to be inactive, which is a fancy way of saying that you hardly move your body at all. (Going from the classroom to the lunchroom to the bathroom to your couch at home hardly counts as physical activity, unless you're walking or biking to school.) Teens today spend more time in front of the TV and the computer than they do moving their bodies, but if you're inactive, it probably isn't completely your fault. You spend a lot of time at school, and these days 92 percent of middle schools and 98 percent of high schools *don't* require daily physical education for students. In addition, increased school workloads, stress, and longer school hours mean that, after a long, hard day, all you might want to do is veg out with comfort food, not exercise for an hour and eat vegetables!

fast fact

The word *gymnasium* comes from the Greek term *gymnos*, which means "naked." In the first gyms of ancient Greece over 2,500 years ago, men exercised in the nude as they trained for athletic competitions!

fast fact

If you're like the average American, you spend nearly five hours a day in front of the television, and that's not including computer time! Couldn't you use a little of that time to get some exercise, even if it's while you're watching TV?

When you're inactive, you might think that you're conserving your energy, but not moving your body actually can make you more tired. You aren't giving your body the metabolism boost it needs to be healthy and burn off extra calories when you don't exercise enough. Because many of us eat way too much and move our bodies way too little, for the first time in history, teens are being diagnosed with what used to be only adult illnesses, including diabetes, high blood pressure, and high cholesterol! Not moving your body may not literally turn you into the rusty, creaky Tin Woodman from *The Wizard of Oz,* but

fast fact

Only 5 percent of mall shoppers use the stairs. However, when a sign promoting the health or size-control benefits of stair climbing is placed near the stairs, usage increases!

a lack of physical exercise can make you feel like him. Physical activity is a big predictor of how healthy we are and how good we feel. Exercise is also a big help in maintaining a healthy size and shape. Even light types of exercise, like walking, tone and tighten your body!

So with all of these benefits, why doesn't everyone exercise enough? Many of us mistakenly believe that exercise has to be painful or difficult to be beneficial, but that is not true!

Are you asking, "With my already overflowing schedule and no gym class at school, how do I make time to exercise?" This chapter shows you not only what to do, but also how to make the most of the few minutes you can spare. It also shows how to move your body in the smallest of spaces, so you have no more excuses! A little exercise is better than nothing. Even going up and down the stairs for only ten minutes is a great way to wake up and start your day! You'll find lots more time-savvy ways to stretch, strengthen, and sweat starting on page 94.

f.y.i.

Don't Overdo It!

WARNING: Yes, you can move your body too much! Most of us will never be in danger of this dilemma, but sometimes it's possible to go overboard and over exercise, especially when we're first starting and are eager to see results! Some of us become "exercise junkies" and our obsession takes a toll on school, work, family, and social relationships. Others overdo it for a little while, hoping to shed a lot of weight quickly. To maintain a healthy body and the right size for your frame, you want to find the level of physical activity that works not just for a brief period but for your entire lifetime. A couple of weeks of exercising crazily might help you shed a couple of sizes fast, but you'll burn out just as quickly, and the stress isn't good for your body. Too much exercise can even lead to a disorder, so see page 159 to make sure you're not overdoing it!

BTW:

COMMON EXCUSES FOR
NOT MOVING YOUR BODY

Are you using any of these excuses to keep from exercising? If so, read on to figure out what is holding you back so that you can get started on getting healthy!

- I don't know how. (That's what this book is for! See page 94 to get started.)
- I don't have enough time. (There's always enough time. See page 162 for ways to juggle your schedule around.)
- I can't afford the equipment I need. (You don't need any equipment! See pages 105–136 for exercises that require nothing but yourself.)
- I have no energy because I'm dieting. (Stop dieting and start filling your body with healthy food! See page 166 for more on feeding your body.)
- I'm too ashamed. (You can exercise in private as well as you can in public! All of the exercises on pages 105–136 are just as effective whether done alone in your room or with a group.)

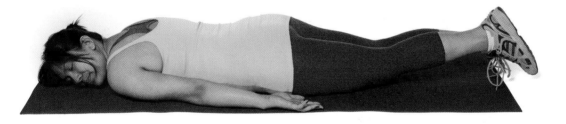

WHY SHOULD I MOVE My Body?
Instead of Just Eating Less?

Exercise makes your body happy and turns it into a calorie-burning machine. Eating too little stresses your body, making it hold onto calories as hard as it can!

Do you remember those confusing "energy in, energy out" equations from the start of the book?

Energy in > Energy out = Our bodies gain weight

Energy in < Energy out = Our bodies lose weight

Energy in = Energy out = Our bodies stay the same weight

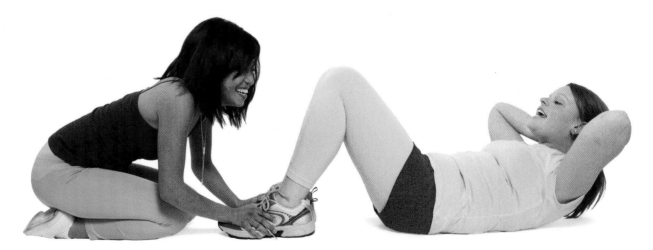

Let's look at what they mean. Calories are a measure of the energy in food. The only way to change the amount of "calories in" is to change the types and quantity of the foods you eat. All foods contain different amounts of energy, and the more of them you eat, the more calories you take in. (More on this in the next chapter.)

Your "calories out" is commonly referred to as "calories burned," and this number comes from a combination of bodily functions, everyday activities, and exercise. Your body uses food energy ("burns calories") to power everything you do, from breathing to carrying your bookbag to biking.

You've probably heard the word *metabolism* before, and while it sounds like something you might keep in a cage and feed insects, it's not! Your metabolism is the rate at which you burn the calories that come from your food every day. Different factors affect the speed of your metabolism. Women usually have slower metabolisms than men, and teens usually have faster metabolisms than adults. However, the two most important factors that affect your metabolism are what you eat and how much you move.

When you don't eat enough or you eat mostly processed, junk, and fast foods that aren't very nutritious, your metabolism slows down, telling your body to hold on to every single calorie that it can because it's not getting the nutrients it needs. A slowed metabolism makes shaping up and getting healthy hard. However, when you combine eating the right amount of healthy food for your activity level and health goals (page 178) with moving your body often by stretching, strengthening, and sweating, your metabolism immediately and excitedly takes note and speeds up, allowing your bodily functions and everyday movements to burn energy instead of conserving it in the form of fat. Exercise also builds lean body tissue—muscle!—which requires more calories to maintain than the body fat it replaces, further increasing your metabolism!

BTW:
FEEL THE BURN!

We say "burn energy" but the proper term is "oxidize." Most (but not all) of the energy our bodies use is converted to a useable form through a series of chemical reactions that use oxygen to break down the body's main fuel, glucose. The process is oxidation, but "burn" sounds more fun, don't you think? I can imagine myself in an exercise class saying, "Let's burn some calories!" but "Let's oxidize some glucose!" just doesn't sound right!

BTW:

OTHER BENEFITS OF MOVING YOUR BODY

In addition to the benefits mentioned earlier, exercise also:

- strengthens bones and muscles
- reduces the risk of breast and colon cancer
- reduces the risk of heart disease
- improves digestion
- helps with menstrual cramps
- gives you better posture
- enables you to live longer
- strengthens your immune system
- helps with acne
- decreases bad moods and depression
- and much more!

Have you experienced some exercise benefits you don't see listed here? Visit www.nancyredd.com to tell me!

Exercise is the best way to speed up your metabolism. It revs up your energy burning abilities, making your body a calorie guzzler. In the same way that a car burns gasoline according to how far you drive it, your body burns calories according to how frequently you move it. The more you move your body, the more calories your body burns, and the better you feel.

Couch potatoes, a.k.a. inactive people, regardless of size or shape or eating habits often:

- don't feel well
- get sick often
- feel tired
- become exhausted quickly
- have trouble focusing or concentrating
- can't do much with their bodies
- become cranky and snap at others
- store excess body fat, regardless of how few calories they consume

However, when you stretch, strengthen, and sweat on a daily basis you:

- have higher levels of energy
- sleep better
- are sharper mentally
- can use your body to perform a lot of tasks
- don't tire easily
- store less excess body fat

So while eating better may be part of your plans to slim down, there's no substitute for moving your body!

Fitness Fads Through History

Over 1,600 years ago – The Martial Arts

Old texts show that the Chinese made a connection between physical inactivity and poor health centuries ago. As early as the sixth century, spiritual and community leaders were promoting exercise and creating a variety of exercise routines, including kung fu, a series of fighting-based movements.

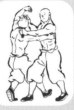

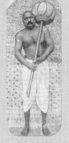

900 years ago – Physical Culture

This form of weight lifting was, and still is, popular in India, with many of the same exercises and equipment still in use today. Unlike Western bodybuilding, which focuses on building big muscles, physical culture emphasizes staying strong in order to perform daily physical tasks. The exercises are designed so that extremely thin people can pack a lot of power.

100+ years ago – Exercise Machines

In the late 1800s, a Swedish doctor created crude versions of what we now know as the StairMaster and Pilates machines, opening up the first machine-oriented gym in Sweden and then building other gyms around the world. The gym memberships were free because the state paid the bill. The market was different in the United States, where rich customers were happy to pay for the

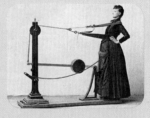

privilege of getting out of the office and sweating a little. Wealthy men and women who could afford to jumped at the chance to try out such novelties as the horse-riding simulator, although many of them owned horses.

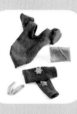

40 years ago – Aerobics

Created in 1968 by a doctor after his own health crisis at age twenty-nine, this exercise method based on getting your heart rate up with cardiovascular exercises or "cardio" training—caught on quickly in the 1970s and 1980s. Aerobics emphasizes such activities as walking, running, cycling, and swimming to build fitness and promote a healthy heart. Aerobic classes are still popular today, though many go by different names. And retro is still rockin' as is evident with Richard Simmons, who started his first fitness facility in 1974 and still teaches aerobics in Los Angeles, always in his 1980s-style fitness attire.

HOW TO   Pick the Perfect Sports Bra

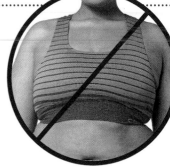

When you are exercising, you need a lot of support—and I don't just mean from your friends and family! While most of us know that we need good gym shoes (see page 152), sports bras are too often overlooked. Wearing no bra or wearing the wrong bra can make your workout harder than it needs to be. When performed in a regular bra, jogging, jumping, and other activities cause breasts to bounce and shift, often in different directions, which can prove uncomfortable, even painful. Don't let that happen to you!

Your sports bra is the most important (and maybe the most expensive, depending upon your chest size) piece of your workout wardrobe, but it's a must for every woman whose cup size is bigger than an AA. Unlike a regular bra, whose only job is to lift and protect during everyday body movements that don't require a lot of effort, such as walking and sitting, a sports bra is designed to comfortably contain and control your breasts when your body is in action. A supportive and comfortable sports bra can be bought from any department store for $15 to $50 (sometimes less if on sale), but as with any other good bra, if you take good care of it (handwashing it in cold water and hanging it to dry) it will last you a long time. Here's what to look for when shopping for a sports bra:

✩ **Are you jiggling?** When you run in place or jump up and down, do your breasts stay comfortably supported or do they bounce this-way-and-that-way inside your shirt? If your breasts are moving around, try a smaller size or a different style.

✩ **Can you breathe?** There is a thin line between snug and suffocating! You want a bra that supports your breasts firmly but does not press uncomfortably around your chest. Once you find one that controls your jiggles, bend over, stretch up and sideways, and breathe deeply to make sure that it's not too tight.

Once you've found the perfect sports bra, buy two! Having a spare ensures that you'll always have a clean, dry one to wear. While the rest of this book focuses on getting healthy as cheaply as possible, if you don't have a good sports bra and shoes, you won't want to exercise, and when you do, you might not move with as much intensity as you should!

Exercise Safety

Now you know WHY you need to move your body, but maybe you don't know HOW. Before beginning any exercise routine, make sure you're not putting your body in danger of injury or overexertion! Don't listen to anyone who tells you "no pain, no gain." While injuries aren't entirely unavoidable (clumsy me, I once broke a toe when a dumbbell slipped out of my hand, which is why I try to stay away from weights), you must do your best to try to stay safe. Here's how:

Always warm up before and after exercise. Take the time. You'll be glad you did. (See page 105 for why.)

Dress properly. You don't have to run out to buy the latest and greatest gear, but you need the essentials. Give your feet—and your boobs—some support.

Start slow. Increase your efforts gradually. If you haven't sprinted in several months, don't dart outside and start running at top speed as soon as your feet hit the ground. That's a sure-fire way to burn out, or worse, hurt something!

Don't push too far. Use the "Talk Test" (page 137) to make sure that you're in the right intensity zone and aren't overdoing anything. You should never feel as if you're going to fall over from exhaustion any second!

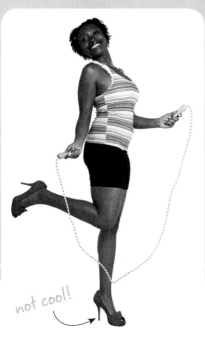

not cool!

Stay hydrated. Drinking water during exercise doesn't cause cramping as some people believe. It does, however, keep you from losing too much fluid, feeling dizzy, or passing out. See page 191 for more on the importance of water.

Listen to your body. If you ever hear something snap, crackle, or pop (aside from your cereal), or you feel the slightest bit of pain, IMMEDIATELY STOP EXERCISING AND TELL SOMEONE, preferably a trainer or a doctor. Exercise injuries often ease up a bit after the initial pain, while they secretly get worse before reappearing in a re-ally bad way. Many won't heal on their own, so don't ignore injuries! Get help from an expert.

HOW CAN I MOVE My Body?

Once you know how to stay safe, you can start figuring out how to move your body for maximal results. While moving your body in any way is wonderful, not all movements are created equal. Ordinary bodily functions like sneezing or blinking can't change your fitness level. Moving your body doesn't mean that you have to rise with the sun and sweat buckets for sixteen hours a day, but neither does it mean that the only exercise you get in a day involves walking from the parking lot into the mall. You should have two goals:

- Give your everyday actions an intensity boost (page 101).
- Get about seven hours of exercise each week, averaging about one hour a day (the exercises on pages 105–137 can help you to fill up this time).

Seven hours may sound like a lot, but it's the minimum amount that a teen girl should be getting in order to stay healthy and grow strong. To get health benefits from exercise, you don't have to do your daily hour all at once. If your schedule is tight, you can break an hour up into shorter time periods and space out your exercise sessions whenever you have some free time.

Some days you may move your body for more than an hour, and some days you may be active for less time (or not at all), but as long as your exercise time totals around seven hours each week, you'll gain all the benefits of exercise, including feeling—and looking—great!

Realistically, however, if you haven't exercised before, you can't immediately start at seven hours a week. You'll need to give your body time to build up its abilities and endurance gradually. So if you think that an hour is too much to start, begin with twenty or thirty minutes a day and gradually build up toward your goal of an hour a day. A little exercise is better than nothing, and we all have to start somewhere!

So what should you do during this daily hour of exercise? There are three main ways to exercise: stretching, strengthening, and sweating. Turn the page to get started on moving your body right away!

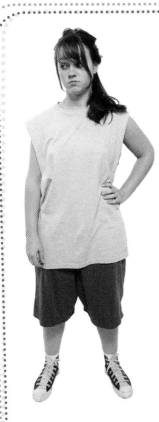

BTW:

FRUMPY FITNESS WEAR

Should you hide your figure flaws under baggy, oversize workout clothes? Probably not! Baggy clothes don't fool anyone; they just make you look frumpy for no reason. Take a look at Chelsea in clothes that overwhelm her, which she chose in an attempt to cover up, versus workout clothes that fit. No matter your size, with a workout wardrobe that skims your body, you'll look much better and you might find exercise easier without all that extra fabric in the way!

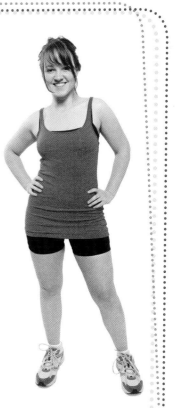

You MOVE Your Body When You . . .
START STRETCHING,
A.K.A. FLEXIBILITY TRAINING

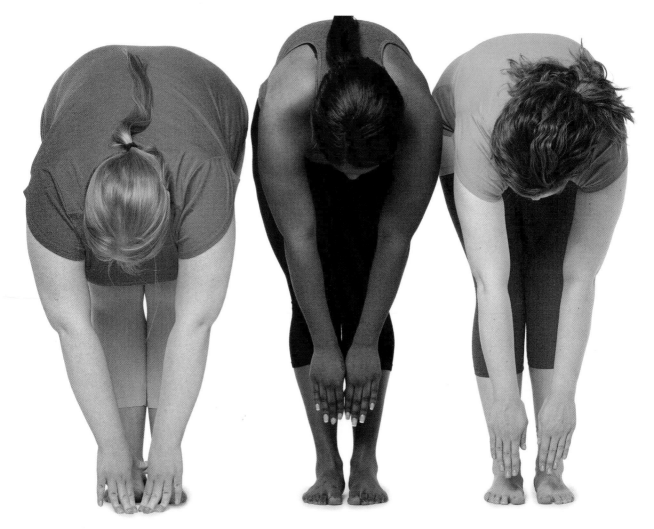

WHAT IS STRETCHING?

Can you bend down and touch your toes? How about your knees? Can you reach the ground without a groan or do you feel as if your body is going to split? Stretching is a good way to improve flexibility. Being flexible means that you can move your muscles and joints in many directions without feeling pain or pressure! Improved flexibility also helps posture, perks up poor moods, and relieves stresses of the body and the mind.

Think of your body as a balloon. When you want to blow up a balloon, you must stretch it first. If you don't it's too stiff to inflate, and might pop if you blow too much air into it! In the same way, many health professionals think that muscles, tendons, and ligaments need a stretch *before* you start your workout. They say that combined with a light warm up (see page 105 for how), pre-exercise stretching lessens the chance of an injury, such as a strain or a sprain. Stretching *after* exercise may help prevent some next-day soreness, too, especially if you are new to exercise. Stretching also helps relieve the pain that commonly comes from hunching over the computer, sleeping in an uncomfortable position, or sitting for long periods of time.

HOW OFTEN SHOULD I STRETCH?

Whether you're going for a walk or off to win a championship game, always stretch for at least five minutes before and after you exercise, using stretches like the ones starting on page 106. Stretching in the form of yoga can count as some of your exercise time. Try the yoga poses starting on page 115 for an hour or two each week—whenever you're stressed or just because they feel good!

Endurance

f.y.i

Although exercise might make you feel fatigued at first, try to keep it up, because the more you get your body used to working up a sweat, the more your endurance builds and your energy level increases. Your improved endurance will let you be active for longer and more intense periods of time without feeling exhausted!

You MOVE Your Body When You...
START STRENGTHENING,
A.K.A. MUSCLE TONING

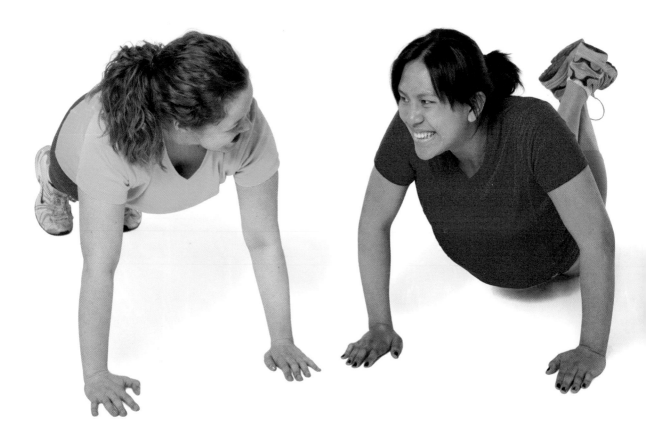

WHAT IS STRENGTHENING?

If your arms were dinosaurs, would they be triceraflops? Do you find yourself fearing heavy doors because you can't push them open without a lot of effort? Can you pick up a heavy suitcase without hurting yourself? Or carry a bursting bookbag without feeling bogged down?

Strengthening your body's muscles (also known as muscle toning or strength training) makes you stronger and more capable of performing daily activities with ease. It's important to strengthen your entire body, from your abdominal muscles (also known as your core) to your arms and legs. Growing stronger is fun, and strengthening your muscles also makes your body look leaner and less jiggly. Even better, strength training is the best way to get results like those you see in ads for too-good-to-be-true diet products. Why? Muscle tissue burns a lot of energy, so increasing your muscle mass means you'll burn more calories even while you sleep!

HOW OFTEN SHOULD I STRENGTH TRAIN?

Try to strengthen and tone for two to three hours each week, regardless of whether you're trying to slim down or just get healthier. Building muscle delivers so many amazing benefits that no one should be without! Don't worry, you don't need fancy machines or dangerous weights to strength train. Turn to page 119 to see how you can grow stronger using nothing but your own body weight.

BTW: RICE

No, not the kind you eat! If you've hurt something while exercising, you MUST see your doctor, but while you're waiting, use the RICE technique to improve the injury:

Rest. Don't put weight on the injured area for forty-eight hours.
Ice. Apply a baggie of ice wrapped in a towel for twenty-minute periods.
Compression. Wear a bandage or an elastic wrap to reduce swelling.
Elevation. Prop the injured body part so that it's higher than your heart to help decrease swelling.

You MOVE *Your Body When You...*
START SWEATING, A.K.A.
CARDIOVASCULAR ENDURANCE

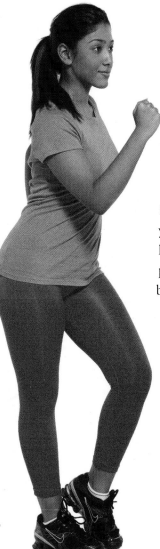

WHAT IS SWEATING?

Can you sprint from your front door to the mailbox and back without feeling as if you're going to collapse afterward? Can you dance until you're drenched with sweat, hardly noticing until the night is almost over?

Working up a sweat through cardiovascular activity ("cardio" for short) is the only way to strengthen the most important muscle in your body, your heart! Cardio clears your mind and lifts your mood, not only strengthening the heart, but also improving lung capacity, increasing energy, and promoting a good night's sleep. Also, cardio's metabolism boost burns off excess body fat, while the act of sweating opens pores and gives your skin a gorgeous, healthy glow, even after you shower off the sweat! You might think that cardio has to happen in public with everyone's eyes on you, but you can also do cardio in the privacy of your own room if you want to, so you have no excuse for not working up a sweat. With cardio, you'll huff, you'll puff, and you'll burn those calories down to the ground!

HOW OFTEN SHOULD I SWEAT?

Aim to do cardio for at least four or five hours every week, especially if you're trying to slim down. While not all cardio turns your T-shirt into a sweatshirt (ha, ha), try to make sure that as much of your cardio as possible has you working up a sweat and barely able to carry on a conversation (see page 137 for more on the "Talk Test"). If you want to work out at home, check out the cardio on page 132 for small-space exercises that enable you to work up a sweat in your bedroom; also check out the chart of other cardio options starting on page 138.

Intensifying Everyday Actions

When you're crunched for time, make the most of every opportunity to boost your metabolism by making your everyday actions more active! The next time you get a chance, try these metabolism-boosting lifestyle changes:

- ✿ Stop riding the elevator and start taking the stairs if your destination is three flights or fewer away from the floor you are on.
- ✿ Park in the first spot that you see instead of driving around looking for a closer parking spot. You'll get more exercise and save gas, too.
- ✿ Do strengthening and stretching exercises while lounging with your laptop or watching television.
- ✿ Pace the room or take a walk when you're talking on the phone instead of staying seated on the sofa.
- ✿ Get off or on public transportation a single stop earlier than usual so that you have to walk a short distance to your destination.

Do you know some great ways to make the most of your day by moving your body more? Visit www.nancyredd.com to share!

FYI: Health Issues and Exercise

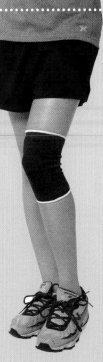

Exercise is all about feeling better and improving ourselves, but no one should make a major change in lifestyle without consulting a professional first. Even if you think you're healthy, talk to your doctor, school nurse, or other health professional about your plans to eat better and exercise more.

That's good advice for all, but it's even more important if you have a medical problem. Be sure to discuss your exercise plans with your doctor if you have:

- an existing or recently healed severe injury (such as a broken bone or multiple stitches)
- asthma or other breathing problems (such as shortness of breath)
- high blood pressure
- known heart trouble
- any problems with your muscles, joints, ligaments, or tendons (such as rheumatoid arthritis)
- an eating disorder
- unexplained weight gain or loss
- a constant feeling of being tired
- dizzy spells
- difficulty sleeping, swallowing, or urinating
- any physical disabilities, whether temporary or permanent (such as a limp)

fast fact

If you have asthma, you're not alone. Nine percent of people under seventeen have it!

belly laughs

BFF#1: You look amazing, girl! What are you doing?
BFF#2: OMG, I stopped eating fast food completely. Also, I watch my calories for two days, and then I skip a day, and then repeat.
BFF#1: That's IT?
BFF#2: Yeah, but it's really hard on the third day. I always worry that I'm not going to make it!
BFF#1: Because you want some fast food?
BFF#2: No, because of the non-stop skipping!

SO,
WHAT ARE YOU WAITING FOR?

Turn the page and get started stretching, strengthening, and sweating today!

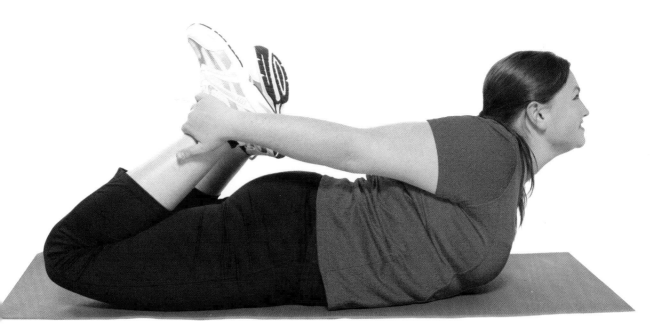

BTW: GYM EQUIPMENT SAFETY

If you're a teen or tween wanting to use gym machines and free weights, don't expect to start pumping iron immediately. Lifting heavy weights can damage your still-growing joints, bones, and tendons, and lifting five- or ten-pound weights should be plenty. Honestly, you don't need to use weights at all if you don't want to! Look at pages 119–131 to find plenty of strength training exercises that don't require weights.

While you don't need machines to make your body strong, if you use exercise equipment such as a treadmill, make sure that you:

☆ **Take an introductory lesson.** Nearly every health club has a staff member or two whose job is to show new members how to use equipment safely. The service is nearly always free. If you can't get a lesson from a pro, consult someone who is experienced for advice. (And, yes, even a "simple" piece of equipment such as a treadmill can be dangerous. I know one girl who fell on a treadmill trying to get off too fast; she ended up needing surgery on both her knee and her shoulder as a result!)

☆ **Read directions.** Jumping on a new exercise machine without the proper instructions is a surefire way to get:

    A. your teeth knocked out.
    B. a concussion.
    C. a weight dropped on a body part.
    D. all of the above.

The answer is D!

☆ **Realize that you, too, can be injured.** Injuries happen to other people. Not you. Right? Wrong. Even if you're fit, going too fast or starting out with too much weight or resistance is guaranteed to give you problems. You might not feel an injury right away, but you could find yourself in serious pain later on.

☆ **Have a spotter on hand close by.** I recommend strength training without weights, but if you're going against my suggestion to strengthen without weights, don't try lifting heavy weights alone. You've seen those funny cartoons of a weight falling on an exerciser's windpipe and he (or she!) is writhing in pain and gagging for air. The situation is not so funny in real life.

ALWAYS WARM UP FIRST!

Before you start stretching, strengthening, or sweating, always take a few minutes to gently wake your muscles. Why? Imagine your body as a string of uncooked spaghetti or a stick of unchewed gum. If you try to bend those things, they snap into pieces! But once you warm them up, they become flexible. Your body is the same way. Once you warm it up, it becomes far more flexible.

So whether you're planning a marathon workout, or trying to squeeze in a quick sweating session, warm up your body first to avoid injuries and make exercising easier. Begin by putting on a playlist or a radio station with upbeat music and for the duration of a song or two (about three to five minutes), march in place to warm up your muscles.

MARCHING IN PLACE

1. Standing up straight with your feet together, lift your knees high, one at a time. You can start off low, but the higher your knees, the more you're warming up your body!

2. Once you're in the groove, start swinging your arms to maximize the movement. When your left knee is raised, your right arm should swing foreword, and vice versa. Keep this up for three to five minutes.

3. To spice up this exercise, move your feet out wider every other minute, keeping your knee lifts high. After a minute, switch back to putting your feet close together, and then go back apart after another minute.

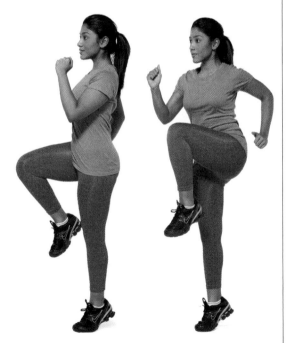

START STRETCHING!
Stretching Before and After Exercise

After your quick warmup, the next step is to stretch your body. Stretching both *before* and *after* exercising reduces the risk of injury and takes a lot of the pain out of strengthening and sweating, and it feels so good! You can stretch standing up, sitting down, or both. I like to start my workout by stretching standing up first, and I cool down with the sitting stretches, but the types of stretches you do and the order you do them in are up to you. Just make sure that you stretch all your body parts and that you hold each stretch for the entire recommended time so that your body gets all the benefits from the stretch!

However you choose to stretch, enjoy how good stretching feels!

STANDING STRETCHES

SHOULDER STRETCH

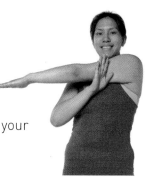

1. Cross one arm across your body toward the opposite side, making sure to keep your elbow straight.

2. Use your other hand or elbow to keep your arm close to your body so that you can feel the stretch.

3. Hold for 20 seconds and then switch sides.

ARM STRETCH

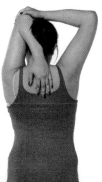

1. As though you have an itch to scratch, lift your right hand and reach behind your head, placing your hand as far down your back as possible.

2. Place your left hand on your right elbow and push gently downward while continuing to reach your right hand down the middle of your back.

3. Hold for 20 seconds and then switch sides.

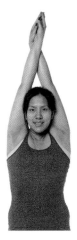

STOMACH AND ARM STRETCH

1. Raise both arms above your head and clap your hands together, crossing your wrists if you can for an extra stretch.

2. Inhale, then while slowly exhaling and keeping your back straight, push your fingertips toward the ceiling and slightly back until you feel the stretch.

3. Hold for 20 seconds and then relax your arms and repeat once.

NECK STRETCH

1. Interlock your fingers behind your head with your thumbs pointing down and your elbows pointing straight ahead.

2. Inhale deeply and, while slowly exhaling, gently try to touch your chin to your chest, keeping your back straight and your shoulders down.

3. Hold for 20 seconds and then relax your hands and repeat once.

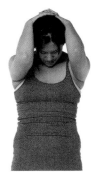

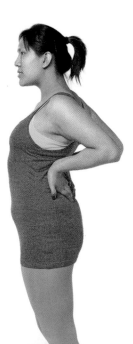

CHEST STRETCH

1. Stand straight with your feet together and, keeping your elbows out to your sides and your fingers pointing downward, place both of your palms against your lower back.

2. Inhale, then exhale slowly and try to get your elbows to touch while keeping your palms steady until you feel the stretch.

3. Hold for 20 seconds and then relax your hands and repeat once.

BACK STRETCH

1. With your feet slightly more than shoulder-width apart and without bending your knees, bend forward and try to touch your toes.

2. Hold for 20 seconds and then, still without bending your knees, try to touch your toes on your right side with both sets of fingers.

3. Hold for 20 seconds and then try to touch your toes on your left side with both sets of fingers. You may try this exercise with your feet closer or farther apart for a different feeling stretch, but do not bounce to try to bend farther because bouncing can strain your muscles.

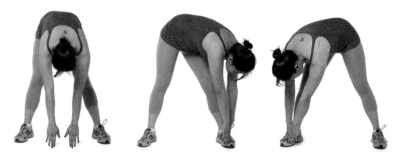

FRONT THIGH STRETCH

1. Standing up straight and keeping your knees together, grasp the top of one foot with your hand. You may need to lean your other hand against a wall or chair for support.

2. Pull your heel toward your tush until you feel the stretch.

3. Hold for 20 seconds and then switch sides.

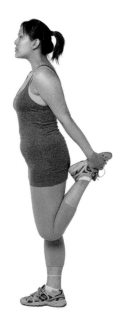

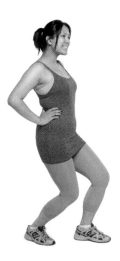

CALF STRETCH

1. Standing up straight with your feet together, place your hands on your hips and move your left foot about a step behind your right foot.

2. Slightly bend your knees while gently pushing your hips forward and dig your left heel into the floor.

3. Hold for 20 seconds and then switch sides.

SHIN STRETCH

1. Standing up straight with your feet shoulder-width apart, bend your right knee slightly and rest both hands on your right thigh. Then move your left foot a half-step in front of your right foot, keeping your back straight and both feet on the floor.

2. Hold for 10 seconds and then point the left foot's toes toward the ceiling while keeping both heels on the floor.

3. Hold for 10 seconds and then switch sides.

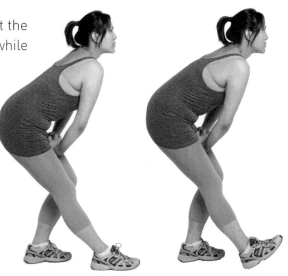

belly laughs

People who are flexible are more easygoing! Their spirits can never be broken and they can never be bent out of shape!

109

FLOOR STRETCHES

TORSO AND TUSH STRETCH

1. Sitting on the floor, straighten your left leg, pointing toes upward, while placing your right foot flat on the floor outside the left knee.

2. Place your left elbow on the outside of your right thigh or knee and turn your head and shoulders to the right, gently pushing your knee downward with your elbow until you feel the stretch.

3. Hold for 20 seconds and then switch sides.

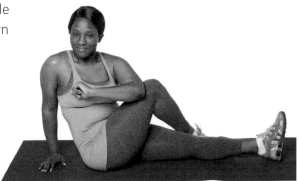

FRONT THIGH STRETCH

1. Lying on your side with your knees and feet together, bend your top leg and grasp the foot.

2. Inhale, then exhale as you gently pull the foot toward your tush.

3. Hold for 20 seconds and then roll over onto your other side and repeat with the other leg and foot.

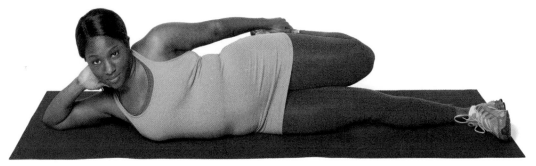

BACK THIGH STRETCH

1. Lying on your back, with both the back of your head and your tush in contact with the floor, grab one leg and straighten it upward, while bending the other knee, taking care to keep your foot on the floor.

2. Get a grip on the calf muscle of the straight leg and try to pull it toward your chest while keeping it straight and your other foot on the floor.

3. Hold for 20 seconds and then switch sides.

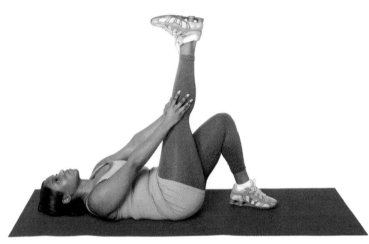

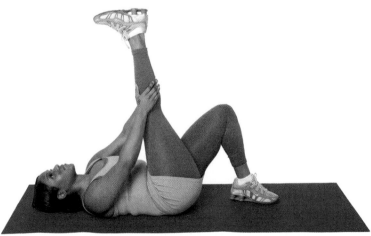

NECK AND SHOULDERS STRETCH

1. Kneel on the floor and extend both hands above your head, fingers pointing forward and touching the floor.

2. Keeping your hands on the floor, face the floor and start pushing your tush back toward your feet until you've made a right angle with the inside of your knee. Push your chest toward the floor so that you can feel the stretch in your neck and shoulders.

3. Hold for 20 seconds and then relax your body and repeat once.

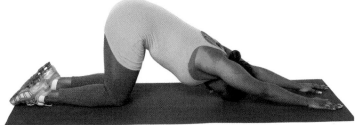

ARM AND BACK STRETCH

1. Kneel on the floor and extend both hands above your head, fingers pointing forward and touching the floor.

2. Keeping your hands on the floor, face the floor and start pushing your tush back toward your feet as far as possible, sitting on your heels if possible. Push your chest toward the floor so that you can feel the stretch.

3. Hold for 20 seconds and then relax your body and repeat once.

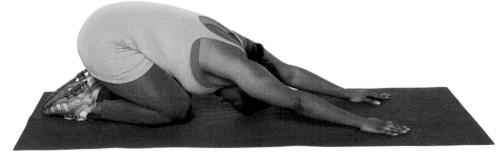

HIP, NECK, AND BACK STRETCH

1. Lying on your back with your knees and feet together, pull both knees to your chest.

2. Gently pull your head as close as you can to your knees.

3. Hold for 20 seconds and then relax your body and repeat once.

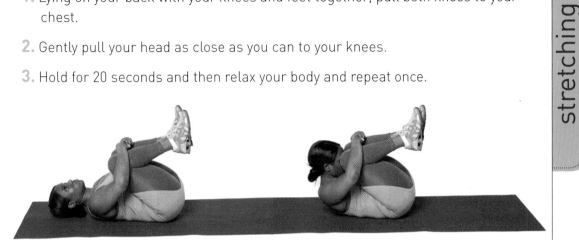

SPINE STRETCH

1. Lying on your stomach with your hands underneath your shoulders and your toe knuckles on the floor, look up toward the ceiling.

2. Inhale, then exhale, straightening your arms and pushing your chest up toward the ceiling with your hands still underneath your shoulders. Clench your tush and make sure your toe knuckles stay on the floor.

3. Hold for 20 seconds and then relax your body and repeat once.

CHEST AND THIGH STRETCH

1. Kneel on the floor and reach backward to grab your heels while pointing your chin to the ceiling.

2. Inhale, then exhale and arch your back, lifting your tush up and forward.

3. Hold for 20 seconds and then relax your body and repeat once.

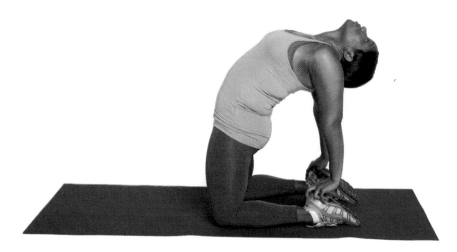

belly laughs

The daughter of a yoga instructor kept getting into trouble at school. Every time her teacher would ask her to do something, she'd agree, but only after turning around and doing a back bend, which made everyone laugh. Finally, she ended up in the principal's office, where she was told that if she didn't do better she would have to be sent home. The next day, her teacher sent her back to the principal's office and she was expelled for three days for disrupting her class. At home, her angry mother asked her what she was doing to get into so much trouble. "I don't know," she cried out. "I've been bending over backward to try and please everyone, just like you told me to!"

KEEP STRETCHING!
Stretching As Exercise Itself

YOGA!

Yoga is very cool, and it is an amazing way to start your day or to begin or end your workout. While yoga is a series of specific poses, you don't have to worry about looking stupid or having poor form. Yoga doesn't have to be perfect! Simply getting started is a huge step. As you get more interested in yoga, consider taking a class or two with a professional who can help you improve your poses!

Before trying the series of poses on the next page called "Sun Salutations," it's best to start with a quick stretch:

BUTTERFLY STRETCH

1. Sitting on the floor with the soles of your feet together, place your hands on the tops of your feet and push your knees toward the floor while keeping your back straight and your hands on your feet.

2. Gently raise your knees and lower them back to the floor ten times, like a butterfly's wings.

3. Rest and repeat once.

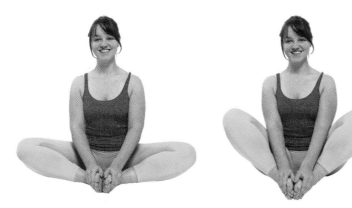

Now let's do some yoga!

115

SUN SALUTATIONS

Each of the twelve poses in a Sun Salutation should be coordinated with your breath, and the set of movements is designed to invigorate your entire body, making you strong, increasing your flexibility, and waking you up from head to toe! People can do Sun Salutations in many different ways, and here's one example:

1. Stand straight and tall in Mountain pose with your palms together in front of your chest, fingers pointing to the ceiling. Inhale and exhale several times.

2. Inhale and, keeping your palms together, raise your arms to the ceiling. If you feel comfortable, arch your back a little and bend backward.

3. Exhale and bend forward touching your hands to your feet, calves, or knees (however far down you can go).

4. Inhale and lunge, stepping your right leg behind you. Place your hands on either side of your left leg, and arch your back.

5. Exhale and step your left leg back to join your right leg and carry your weight on your feet and hands for Plank pose. Inhale.

6. Exhale and lower your knees, then your chest and forehead, pushing your hips up and keeping your toes curled under.

7. Inhale, straighten your arms, uncurl your toes, and stretch your upper body forward, pushing your hips down and puffing your chest out as you bend your back and look up at the ceiling for Upward Dog pose.

8. Exhale and recurl your toes to lift your hips to the ceiling while pressing your heels down to the floor for Downward Dog pose.

9. Inhale and lunge again, bringing your right leg forward and placing your hands on either side of your right leg.

10. Exhale and bring your left foot forward while bringing your head down to your knees and touching your hands to your feet, calves, or knees (however far down you can go).

11. Inhale and, keeping your palms together, raise your arms to the ceiling. If you feel comfortable, bend your back a little as described above.

12. Exhale and bring your palms together in front of your chest, with your fingers pointing to the ceiling, standing straight and tall in Mountain pose. Inhale and exhale several times.

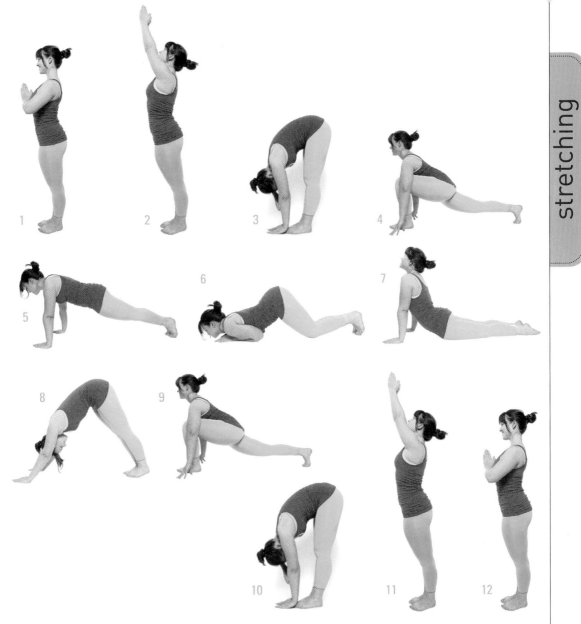

On your second set, switch sides and step back with your left leg. Begin slowly so that you master each pose, and then you can work your way up to a continuous series of motion. With practice, your body will know just what to do the moment your feet hit the floor! Once you've mastered sun salutations, speed up a bit and do multiple repetitions for an amazing exercise. When you breathe and pose properly, a sped-up sun salutation can get your heart pumping, so give it a shot!

I CONFESS:
YOGA CHANGED MY LIFE!

Aside from cheerleading, I never found a sport or group activity that I enjoyed until my senior year in college. When I told a friend that I was trying to get in shape, she suggested I come with her to a yoga class. I immediately declined. Wasn't yoga either for very thin, rich people, or else for hippies? Wouldn't I look ridiculous? I didn't want to go because I didn't think that I would like it and because I couldn't figure out how a bunch of stretches would help me shape up.

Thank goodness my friend wouldn't take no for an answer! As soon as I opened the door to the yoga classroom, most of my worries vanished. People of all shapes, sizes, ages, and lifestyles were there. They weren't dressed to impress; they wore comfortable clothing. I instantly felt as if I belonged, but my confidence crashed again after stumbling on the very first pose and quickly falling behind everyone, including the eighty-year-old in front of me who put my moves to shame!

Luckily, the teacher saw my frustration and impatience and took extra time to position my body and to help me breathe properly. Each time the teacher corrected me, I'd instantly feel how the change affected my body for the better; by the end of the hour, I wasn't as awesome as the eighty-year-old, but I was doing pretty well and, most important, I felt amazing. I incorporated yoga into my exercise schedule and it gave me the confidence I needed to go after my goal of competing in the Miss Virginia Pageant. My posture improved, my body felt longer and taller, and my mind and soul felt happier, too. Even today, when I'm feeling stressed, a little yoga calms my mind and invigorates my body. Yoga helped me learn how to control my body, and it taught me to not let my fears and unfounded opinions stand in the way of self-improvement. Maybe the poses on page 115–117 will change your life for the better, too!

START STRENGTHENING!
Strengthening Your Core

Toning up your tummy is more than a great way to get rid of rolls. Working your core can have some impressive health benefits! Your core is more than just your abdomen; it includes your back and tush. Your core controls your posture, and it helps you move your body more efficiently and easily, whether you're exercising or performing everyday actions. Try to keep your stomach sucked in while working your core, but don't forget to breathe. A fun way to visualize this action is to imagine pulling your belly button in to touch your spine.

Different types of core exercises work the muscles in different ways, so don't feel as if you need to stick to plain old crunches!

CHAIR KNEE LIFTS

You can do these while you're watching television or while you're waiting for something to download on your computer!

1. Sitting on the edge of your chair, grab the sides of your chair for balance, lean back a little bit, and bend your knees.

2. Pull your belly button toward your spine and pull your knees toward your chest using only your stomach muscles and not your arms.

3. Slowly lower your feet almost to your starting position, but when they're about to touch the floor, raise your knees back up to your chest. Each knee lift counts as one repetition of this core exercise.

4. Repeat at least 10 times in a row and work your way up to 20 or 30 repetitions.

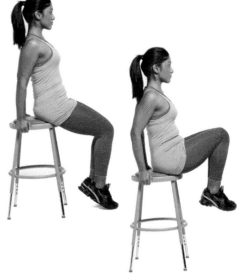

PLANK

This is a great core exercise. You'll feel it, and you'll be proud of yourself as you grow strong enough to hold the position for a longer period of time.

1. Lying on your stomach, make fists with your hands and rest your elbows and forearms on the floor underneath your shoulders.

2. Pull your belly button toward your spine, tighten your tush, and push your hips off the floor until you are raised up onto your toes and your forearms. Don't forget to breathe!

3. Try to keep your back flat and your body as straight as possible for at least 10 seconds. Build up until you can hold the position for up to 60 seconds at a time.

4. Rest for 15 seconds and repeat 3 times.

TORSO TWISTS

Whittle your waist with this easy yet effective exercise!

1. Stand up straight with your feet flat on the floor and bring your arms up into a muscle stance.

2. Pull your belly button toward your spine and rotate your torso from left to right, pivoting your feet and knees in the direction that you're twisting your torso. Each time you twist both left and right counts as one repetition.

3. Repeat at least 10 times. Work your way up to 20 or 30 repetitions.

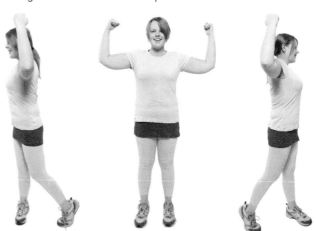

BACK EXTENSIONS

Move over, muffin top! This simple squeeze will help you get rid of back bulges and makes you stronger. So bring on the heavy backpack!

1. Lying on your stomach with your legs extended straight out and your feet together, place your hands behind your neck.

2. Pull your belly button toward your spine, inhale, then exhale, slowly lifting your head and chest off the floor, in a backward crunch toward your tush, while keeping your hips and legs straight and immobile. You don't need to lift your chest off the floor very far to feel this exercise.

3. Inhale while slowly lowering your chest back down to the floor. One chest lift counts as one repetition.

4. Repeat at least 10 times in a row, and work your way up to 20 or 30 repetitions.

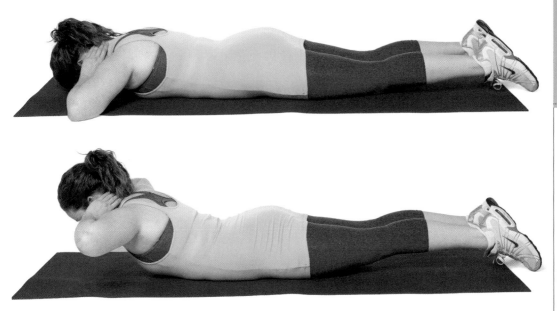

REVERSE CRUNCH

Try this variation on this popular abdominal exercise for a change of pace!

1. Lying on the floor with your arms at your sides, palms down, raise your legs to the ceiling, bend your knees slightly, and cross your ankles.

2. Pull your belly button toward your spine and lift your hips off the floor toward the ceiling while keeping your palms on the floor. Hold for one or two seconds before bringing hips back down to the floor.

3. Repeat 10 times, and work your way up to 20 or 30 repetitions.

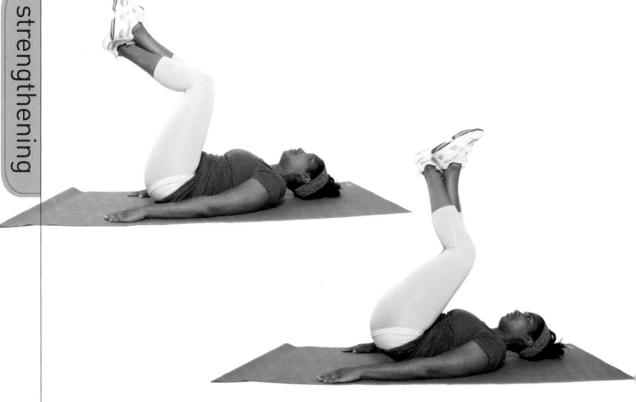

strengthening

CRUNCHES

If you're more comfortable working your core with crunches, add a side twist to spice things up!

1. Lying on the floor, bend your knees and place your hands behind your head or across your chest while keeping your feet flat on the floor, shoulder-width apart.

2. Looking up at the ceiling and keeping a space between your chest and your chin, inhale, then exhale and raise your chest toward your knees until your shoulders lift off the floor.

3. Inhale and lower your shoulders back to the floor. Exhale and rotate your chest toward one side, then inhale and lower your shoulders back to the floor. Alternate sides. Each time you twist center, left, and right counts as one repetition.

4. Repeat at least 10 times in a row, and work your way up to 20 or 30 repetitions.

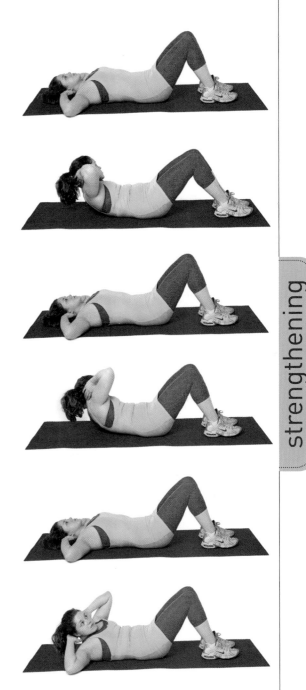

KEEP STRENGTHENING!
Strengthening Your Arms and Legs

Your core isn't the only body part that could stand to get stronger. These easy exercises will tone and tighten your arms and legs! You'll appreciate your enhanced strength whether you're taking on a sweating session or a shopping spree.

BICEP TOWEL PULL

You can tone up anytime, even right after your shower using nothing but a towel!

1. Twist a large towel into a long rope. Step on one end of the roped towel with your left foot and grab the other end with your left hand. Keep your right hand by your side and your feet slightly apart.

2. Pull the towel up toward the ceiling until you feel a pull in your upper arm. Hold for 20 seconds. Don't forget to breathe while pulling the towel! Switch sides.

3. Each time you pull both left and right sides counts as one repetition. Repeat 3 times with 15-second rest periods between the repetitions.

4. Work your way up to holding this position for 60 seconds at each repetition.

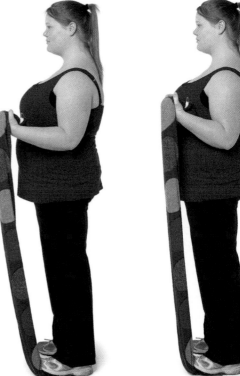

SHOULDER TOWEL HOLD

While these movements may seem small, they make a big difference. You will definitely feel the results afterward!

1. Twist a large towel into a long rope. Step on one end of the roped towel with your left foot and grab the other end with your left hand. Keep your right hand by your side and your feet slightly apart.

2. Holding your towel, pull your arm out to your side until you feel a pull in your shoulder. Hold for 20 seconds. Don't forget to breathe while pulling the towel! Switch sides.

3. Each time you pull both left and right sides counts as one repetition. Repeat 3 times with 15-second rest periods between the repetitions.

4. Work your way up to holding this position for 60 seconds with each repetition.

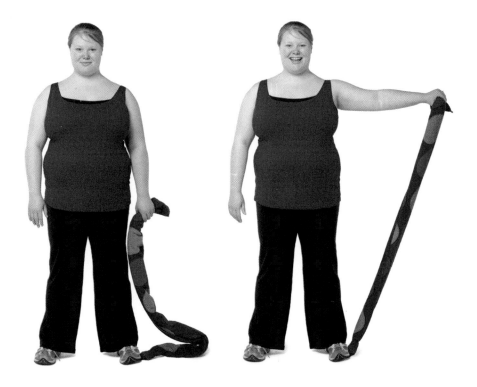

strengthening

SWIMMING

Just as actual swimming does, this exercise strengthens your core as well as your arms and legs.

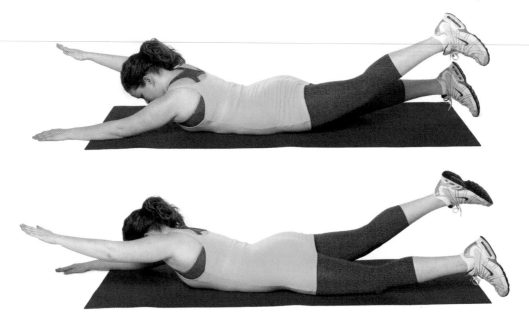

1. Lying on your stomach with your eyes facing the floor, pull your belly button toward your spine and extend your legs and arms slightly above the floor.

2. Raise your right arm and left leg slightly higher for one second, then switch to raising your left arm and right leg. Raising both your right and left arm counts as one repetition. Repeat at least 10 times; then rest for 15 seconds.

3. Work your way up to 20 or 30 repetitions. Try not to let your legs and arms touch the floor until you finish all your repetitions.

REVERSE PLANK

While the plank exercise is excellent for strengthening your core, the reverse plank is great for your entire body!

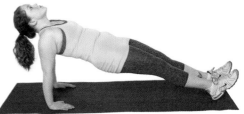

1. Sit on the floor with your arms by your sides and your palms touching the floor. Look up at the ceiling.

2. Pull your belly button toward your spine and squeeze your tush and thighs, pushing up onto your heels and palms into a reverse plank. Try to keep your back flat and your body as straight as possible for at least ten seconds. Repeat 3 times with 15 seconds of rest between the repetitions.

3. Work your way up to holding this position for 60 seconds.

TRICEP LIFTS

You don't have to lie down to do this exercise. You can do it standing or sitting on a backless chair.

1. Lying on your stomach with your eyes facing the floor, place your arms at your side with your palms up.

2. Pull your belly button toward your spine and raise your arms toward the ceiling as

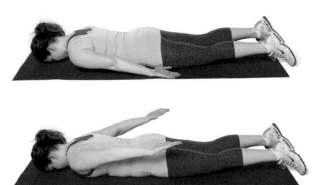

high as you can while keeping your thighs touching the floor. Hold for 2 seconds before lowering back down to the floor. Repeat 10 times.

3. Rest for 15 seconds and then do 10 more. Work your way up until you can complete 20 or 30 repetitions.

PUSH-UPS

As you get stronger, it might not take you long to progress from the modified version to the full push-up!

Modified Push-ups

1. Kneeling on your hands and knees, face downward, making sure that your knees are hip-width apart and your hands are just above and slightly wider than your shoulders. Keep your toes touching the ground throughout this exercise.

2. Inhale, pull your belly button toward your spine and, upon exhaling, bend your elbows and lower your chest as close to the floor as possible. Inhale again and straighten your arms, bringing your chest back up.

3. Repeat at least 5 times in a row, and work your way up to 20 or 30 repetitions. Don't forget to breathe!

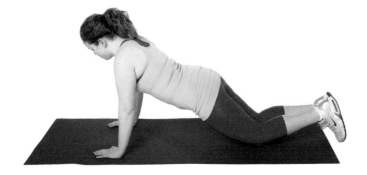

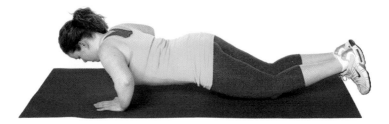

Regular Push-ups

Once you build up your strength, these regular push-ups really pack a punch!

1. With your toes and your palms touching the floor, face downward, making sure that your feet are hip-width apart and your hands are just above and slightly wider than your shoulders.

2. Inhale, pulling your belly button toward your spine and, upon exhaling, bend your elbows and lower your chest as close to the floor as possible. Inhale again and straighten your arms, bringing your chest back up.

3. Repeat at least 5 times. Work your way up to 20 or 30 repetitions. Don't forget to breathe!

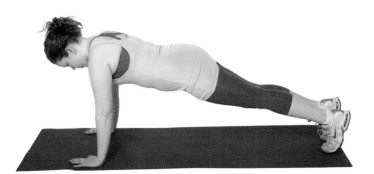

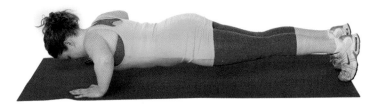

Simple Swaps for Expensive Workout Gear

Skipping around with a piece of string in your hands might seem a little silly, but if no one is around to see you, who cares? Here are some household items that can serve as great replacements for expensive exercise equipment.

- Soup cans = **one-pound weights**
- Sugar bags = **five-pound weights**
- Water-filled milk jugs = **handled, adjustable weights**

- Clothesline rope = **jump rope**
- Old tights or hose = **strength band**
- Rubber gloves = **weight-lifting gloves**

Got some savvy substitutions that you'd like to share? Visit www.nancyredd.com and tell me about how you save money while getting stronger!

belly laughs

Potato sacks are great for fitness, too! Start off by holding a five-pound potato sack in each hand, standing still for as long as you can. After a while, you can move up to ten-pound sacks, then fifty-pound sacks, and finally, after tons of practice, you should be able to lift hundred-pound sacks in each hand for over a minute! Try it, it really works! Once you get to the hundred-pound sacks, the next step is to try putting a few potatoes in each empty sack, but I tried that and didn't get very far so don't overdo it!

SIDE LEG LIFTS

Tone your thighs in two minutes! Make sure to lift in all directions to work all aspects of the area.

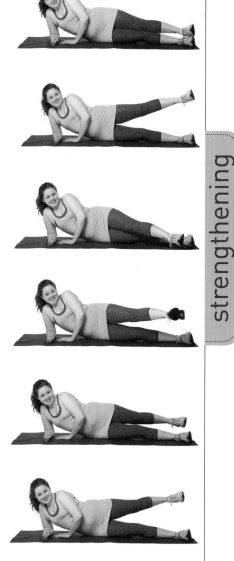

1. Lie on your right side with your feet together, one on top of the other. Prop your upper body up onto your right elbow and face forward, letting your left hand touch the floor in front of your chest.

2. Pull your belly button toward your spine and slowly raise your left leg until it is shoulder height, then lower it back to your body, keeping your toes pointed in the same direction as your eyes.

3. Repeat 10 times and then rest for 10 seconds.

4. Next, raise your left leg in front of your body until it is shoulder height, then lower it back to your body behind your right leg, keeping your toes pointed in the same direction as your eyes.

5. Repeat 10 times and then rest for 10 seconds.

6. Finally, raise your left leg behind your body until it is shoulder height, then lower it back to your body in front of your right leg, keeping your toes pointed in the same direction as your eyes.

7. Repeat 10 times and then rest for 10 seconds.

8. Switch sides and repeat all exercises. Eventually you should be able to increase your repetitions until you're doing 30 in each position!

strengthening

START SWEATING!
Sweating in Small Spaces

While getting outside or doing group exercise is great for you, you can get a good workout in the smallest of spaces! Here are some easy exercises that can have you breaking a sweat and checking off ten, twenty, even thirty minutes of your cardio!

PUNCHES

1. Standing with your feet slightly apart, keep your back flat and bend over slightly so that your chest is parallel to the floor and your body makes a right angle. Your eyes should always be looking ahead.

2. Inhale, then exhale as you extend your right fist forward and your left fist back.

3. Inhale and bring your fists back to your chest.

4. Exhale and switch arms, extending your left fist forward and your right fist back.

5. Repeat, switching arms at a quick pace!

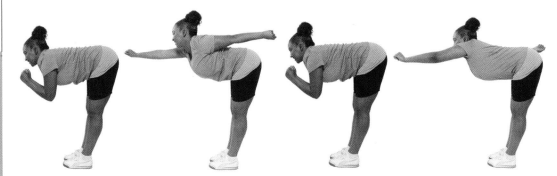

HAMSTRING CURLS

1. Standing straight and keeping your knees shoulder-width apart, make fists and straighten your arms in front of your body.

2. Inhale and pull your elbows back and your fists into your side while lifting your left heel toward your tush as though you're trying to kick your own backside.

3. Exhale and return your arms and feet to the beginning position.

4. Inhale and bring your elbows back and your fists into your side once more while lifting your right heel toward your tush.

5. Repeat, switching feet at a quick pace!

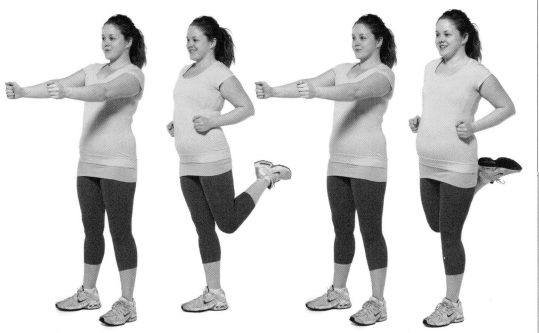

sweating

133

POWER JUMPS

1. Standing straight and keeping your knees together and your hands by your side, squat, keeping your thighs parallel to the floor as though you are trying to sit on an invisible chair.

2. Inhale, then exhale and jump up off the floor with all your might while stretching your arms above your head at the same time.

3. Inhale and return to the squatting position.

4. Repeat at a quick pace!

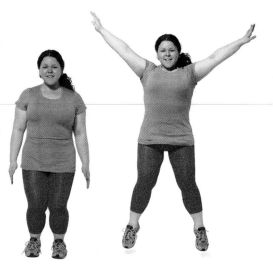

WINDMILLS

1. Standing with your legs out wide, bring your left arm down toward your right foot while extending your right arm behind your body.

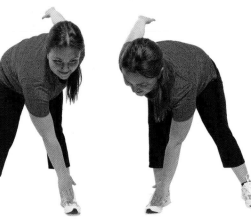

2. Without standing back up, bring your right arm down toward your left foot and extend your left arm behind your body.

3. Repeat, switching arms at a fast pace!

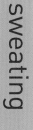

sweating

DANCE PARTY!

1. Put on your favorite music, close your door, and just start jamming! Invite some friends over, use your hairbrush as a microphone, and get your heart rate up while having fun!

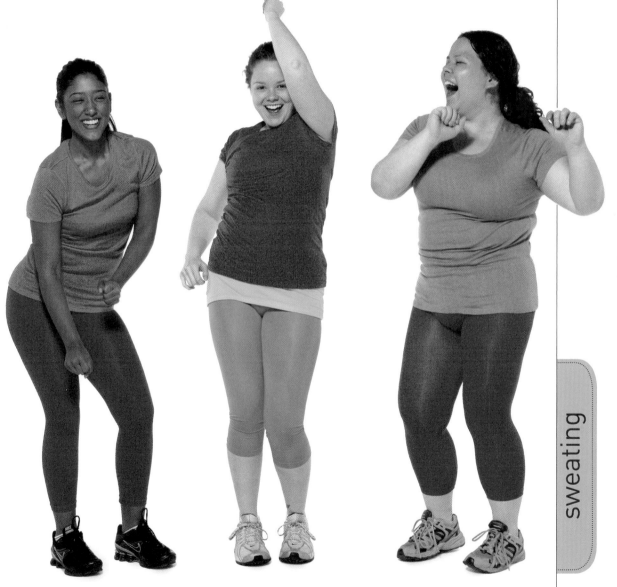

Other Cardio that Costs Nothing

There's not enough room in this book for all the cardio options available to you, but here are a few simple, private, and FREE ways to move your body that will have you fit in no time!

☆ **Running or walking the stairs.** For the average 135-pound person, running up and down the stairs can burn as much as 150 calories or more in only ten minutes! Just be sure to hold the rail (wear a glove to protect from friction burns) and watch your step. If you are afraid of a fall, walking the steps at a fast pace still provides a solid cardio workout.

☆ **Housecleaning.** Scrubbing, vacuuming, mopping, and sweeping are more strenuous than they seem, burning around 175 calories in an hour for a 135-pound person. Plus, afterward you have the added bonus of a clean house!

☆ **Borrowing fitness DVDs.** If you want to spice things up, look to your local library, which probably lends dozens of exercise routines from celebrity trainers for free. If you can't wait, look online for workout programs, which can help you burn anywhere from 100 to 400 calories per hour!

What's your favorite cardio workout? Visit www.nancyredd.com to share your ideas and also to find a list of fun, free routines to look for online!

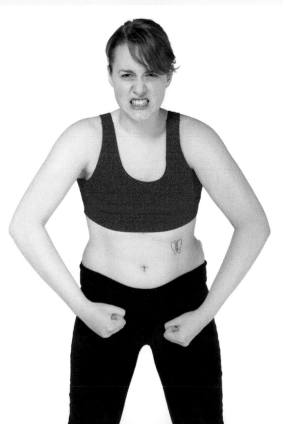

fast fact

If you're working out hard but sweating only a little, you might be dehydrated. Check page 201 for ways to drink more water.

HOW TO Use the Talk Test to Measure Exercise Intensity

While any cardio is excellent exercise, you should vary the intensity level of your cardio workouts depending on your fitness goals. Intensity means how hard you're working. If you are trying to slim down or improve your fitness or endurance levels, try to make your workout more intense than if you're only trying to maintain good health. At the same time, you don't want to overdo it: You could strain a muscle or end up too sore to start again the next day, which does you no good.

The "Talk Test" is a fun and easy tool for determining the intensity of your exercise. Here's how to do it:

Step 1) Start moving. After warming up and stretching (see page 105), get going for a few minutes at a slow pace, then slowly ramp up to the rate that you think makes the most sense for you.

Step 2) Try to talk. The right intensity, which is about when you start to sweat from the activity (and not the weather), should make you feel a bit breathless. You should find talking a little difficult, but not impossible. You can talk to yourself, to someone next to you, or, as I love to do, on the phone using a hands-free device.

Step 3) Adjust the intensity of your exercise if you need to. If talking is impossible, you're probably exercising too intensely to be safe or healthy, so drop down a notch! But if you can gab away easily, up your intensity to get more out of your workout.

If you want to decrease your intensity, go slower, and lower your knees and drop your arms to your sides while walking or running. If you want to increase your intensity, go faster, raise your knees higher and pump your arms and legs more while walking or running.

WARNING: Never go too far too fast. The "Talk Test" will help you avoid getting to the point where you're breathing so hard for so long that you feel weakened, dizzy, or faint. That's not normal, healthy, or helpful to your long-term goals of looking and feeling great! For more on how to avoid feeling bad after a workout, turn to page 152.

KEEP SWEATING!
Sweating Anywhere

Many different fun activities count as exercise when you get a good sweat going. Some are fun and easy to do instantly, while others require practice. You might not like some or even be very good at them, but one thing is certain: You'll never know unless you try! Whether you get into a group or solo sport or try an active hobby on your own or with a team, the possibilities are endless, so check out this list of exercise options. If something interests you, look for opportunities in your hometown.

kickboxing	track and field	volleyball
ice-skating	bicycling	hiking
swimming	golf	mall walking
aerobics	horseback riding	jumping rope
salsa dancing	softball	Frisbee
rock climbing	rollerblading	marching band
pilates	hockey	skateboarding
karate	basketball	roller skating
Gymnastics	Tae Bo	Tae kwon do
cheerleading	soccer	hip hop dancing
spinning	tennis	football
	racquetball	

Got a favorite activity that you don't see here? Visit www.nancyredd.com to share!

I CONFESS: I RIDE A TRIKE!

Talk about embarrassing! One of my deepest secrets (until now) is that I walk on my toes most of the time because of a medical issue. Walking that way is not painful or problematic for me; in fact, it's an advantage when it comes to walking in high-heeled shoes. However, because of my condition, I'm clumsy and my balance is poor (which is why I love yoga so much; it improves balance). Astrology-wise, I'm a Taurus, so I really am like a bull in a china shop! For those reasons, I'm wary of riding anything with wheels and pedals, as I can easily tip over and have done so in the past. When I was a kid, I had a horrible bike accident that ruined my entire summer (and permanently scarred my leg), so ever since then I've steered clear from what was once one of my favorite forms of entertainment.

When I moved to the beach recently, I became jealous of all the normal-footed bikers with their hair blowing in the wind, cruising along without a care in the world. But I wasn't envious enough to risk my life, so I chalked cycling up as an experience I could never have again. When Christmas came, my guy surprised me with a present I didn't know existed—an adult tricycle. It is a little bit bigger than a regular bicycle, but the support of the extra wheel keeps me steady. Sure, I get some funny stares sometimes, but because biking is one of the few cardio exercises that I truly enjoy, I can tolerate a few stares as I ride happily by the ocean every day just like everyone else in Santa Monica.

Having a physical limitation can be a challenge, but there are options that can make things work for you and your circumstances. I learned with my trike that a little creativity can go a long way!

HOW TO Power Walk

A few small changes can make a big difference in the intensity of your cardio workout. For example, you can turn regular walking into power walking, increasing the calories burned in an hour of walking (for a 135-pound person) from 250 to over 400. Here's how.

Step 1) When power walking, posture is everything. While relaxing your shoulders, keep your back straight, your butt tight, your stomach sucked in, and your chest raised. Your eyes should always be looking forward. Even if you're power walking with a friend and want to chat, learn to talk without looking at your friend's face.

Step 2) Walking in a straight line, take small, fast steps that push off with your toes and land on your heels. A natural bounce will occur and help you move faster!

Step 3) Bend your arms at the elbow to almost a ninety-degree angle and curl your hands into loose fists. Staying in rhythm with your feet and keeping your arms close to your sides, start swinging your arms from the elbow only, front to back, like a rocking chair. Don't cross or swing your arms from left to right. And don't let your arms cross your chest.

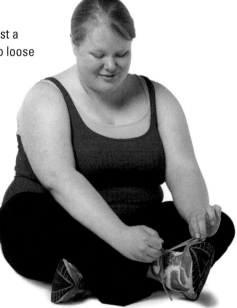

Step 4) Breathe naturally and deeply, but don't overdo it. Using the "Talk Test," you should be able to carry on a conversation (though it might be a winded one), which makes power walking the perfect workout to share with friends!

BTW: INJURWIIS

Game systems such as the Wii can help kickstart a couch potato's exercise routine, but as with any type of exercise, "InjurWiis" (or "Wiinjuries," call them what you want) are no laughing matter. Recent studies have found that, while on average kids burn about 150 calories per hour playing Wii Fit, more than 10 percent of players experience frequent finger and wrist pain. Emergency rooms report Wii-inflicted black eyes, bruised knees, and foot fractures. While no official studies have been done in America yet, Britain reports ten Wii-related hospital visits per day!

You can avoid Wii-itis and having to go into Wiihab from your electronic exercise by using common sense and treating the Wii like any other form of exercise. Warm up beforehand, taking care to stretch your arms and fingers. Clear enough space to move around safely, give your body a break every now and then between games, drink lots of water before, during, and after playing, and keep a firm grip on your controller so it doesn't go flying out of your hand and Wiinjure you or someone else!

fast fact

In 1991, a rookie with the Sacramento Kings team of the National Basketball Association allegedly missed two games because he developed tendonitis in his right wrist from playing too many video games! Remember, no one is above injury!

Counterfeit Calorie Counts

f.y.i.

Have you noticed the calorie counter display that's built into many pieces of exercise equipment? It can read too high or too low by as much as 30 percent! The exerciser's height, weight, and body position—even factors such as room temperature—can increase or decrease the reading, meaning the number you see there is merely a guess. Outside a laboratory, there's no way to make an accurate measurement of calories burned, but knowing the exact number of calories burned is not nearly as important as knowing that you are exercising at the right intensity level and for an hour a day, so worry more about making time to workout than the probably-wrong numbers on the machines! You can estimate the intensity of your exercise if you use the "Talk Test" (see page 137 for a how-to).

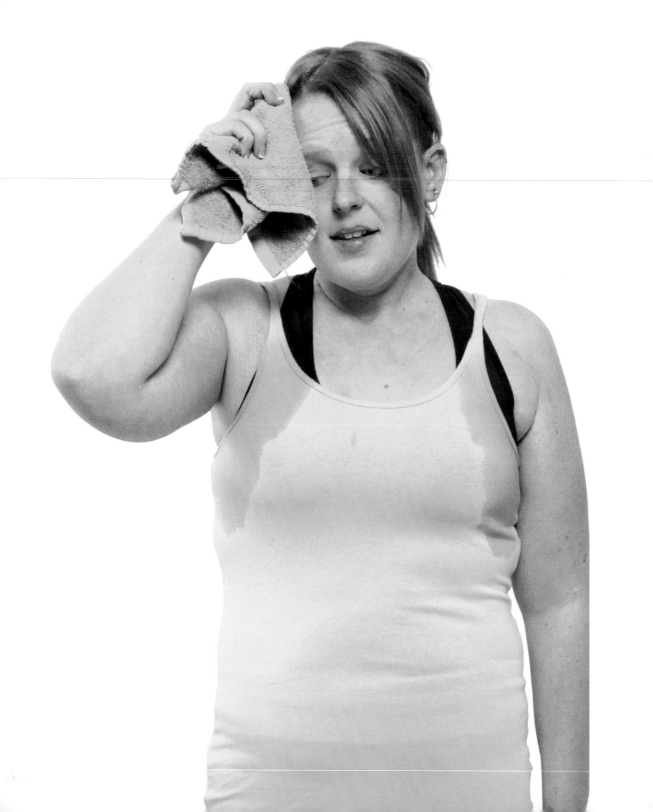

Move Your Body
DRAMAS

I exercise a lot but I still don't look "fit."

WHAT'S GOING ON?

It's a fact: Real women have curves, and while Barbie's abs are made of rock-hard plastic, that's not how nature made yours! Women are built to have more body fat than men. (The body weight of an average normal-weight man is 15 percent fat; a woman's is 25 percent.) Women have more fat cells in their bodies, too—about 9 billion more (26 billion for men and 35 billion for women). Fat storage is no accident. It's nature! We need those curves and extra fat cells to menstruate properly and, eventually, to have babies. While exercise is excellent at helping you tone, trim, and look and feel amazing, most women, muscular or not, tend to have a soft layer of fat underneath their skin that won't disappear easily, if at all.

But before you get frustrated and scrap your exercise plans, know that getting washboard abs and weighing less aren't always the most important things, even if you're trying to get fit! Exercise won't always make you lose weight, especially if you're already at a healthy size for your age and height. In fact, as you become more fit, you might gain weight! Exercise makes you strong and increases the size of your muscles, which weigh more than fat. When heavier but sleek-looking muscle takes the place of light but lumpy-looking excess fat, the scale sometimes goes up instead of down, even if you're looking better. So though you might not see a muscle sticking out, it's there, and it shows itself in how much stronger you become!

HOW DO I DEAL?

If you're averaging seven hours of exercise a week, you're doing exactly what you should to get your body into tiptop shape, so stop feeling "fat" because you can pinch a layer of body fat under your skin! Your body needs that layer. In fact, your period can stop if your body fat dips too low. While getting rid of periods might sound like a relief, you won't be healthy if you stop having them!

If you're worried about the wiggles and you're already sweating four or five hours a week with cardio, try increasing your strength training so you build more muscle. If you are trying to slim down some and aren't seeing results, turn back to page 42 and check out the many ways that you can see if you're moving toward your goals. Pay particular attention to your measurements, which are a better gauge of how well you're doing than your weight is—miniuscule measurement changes can add up over time! But remember: Although getting in shape is an awesome goal, try not to take exercise to the extreme. Just because the models look ripped in the magazines doesn't mean their butts are truly rock hard. The photographs you see in magazines have been digitally altered. Some of those models have painted on— yes, PAINTED ON!—abs.

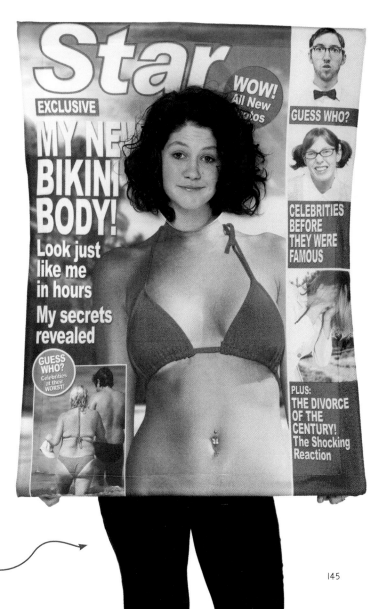

We can't walk around with our head stuck in a blown-up magazine cover!

I CONFESS:
MY BOYFRIEND MADE FUN OF MY FLAB!

"BWEH BWEH BWEH! BWEH BWEH BWEH!" My boyfriend's hands were on my love handles, but all I could feel was hate as I screamed back, "OMG, dude, for the last time, STOP doing that." He wouldn't stop jiggling my stomach and making funny noises anytime the mood struck him, regardless of whether anyone else was around to see. At the time of the tummy grabs, I had recently worked my way back into great shape, but I was still insecure. Even with countless crunches, I've never been able to build visible ab muscles, not even for the Miss America Pageant! Only months after the relationship ended did I think back and realize that he only started grabbing my stomach after I confided in him that I was worried about the way my abs looked. Instead of consoling me and telling me that my stomach was superb, he made fun of the body part that made me feel most vulnerable.

Although he was super cute (and a great kisser), I finally decided that I deserved better. The next BWEH BWEH BWEH belly moment, I screamed back, "If you BWEH BWEH BWEH me one more time, I'm going to BWEH BWEH BWEH you out of my life!"

He looked shocked and stayed on his best behavior for a little while, until one day, in front of my friends, and right after I'd won a major award, he grabbed my gut and at the top of his lungs shouted BWEH BWEH BWEH. I immediately made good on my promise to dump him and, despite his disbelief and efforts to win me back, I never considered resuming the relationship! I moved on and eventually found someone who loves me and has never said a negative thing about my body.

Looking back, I now realize that making me feel bad about my body made my old boyfriend feel powerful. If you have someone in your life who is constantly teasing or belittling you, it's time to get out of that relationship and find someone who praises you and your body instead of putting you down. I promise: There's someone better out there, just for you, and you don't deserve to be made fun of by anyone, but especially not a romantic partner!

146

Success Story: Patricia

"In my early teens I tried to lose weight with strict dieting. I only exercised off and on. I tried all the popular fad diets, like Atkins, but the hunger and yo-yo dieting messed with my self-esteem and my metabolism. It wasn't until I started working at Curves, a cool gym just for women, that I learned how to eat right AND exercise. I learned that it's not good for our bodies to choose one over the other. I've been working at Curves for six years, and the best thing about my job is that I am paid to be healthy. I am encouraged to eat well, and I never have an excuse to skip exercise. I can't blame work or being too busy because the machines are staring me in the face every single day!

"My biggest lesson has been realizing that BMI is not the right gauge for my personal health. From the outside, I might not look superstrong, but at 5'3" and 146 pounds, I pack a whole lot of muscle. Because BMI doesn't take muscle into account, by its standards I am overweight, which is not true! You can tell from my pictures that I'm not.

"My second biggest body lesson has been realizing that nothing happens overnight. Losing weight and building strength take time, so it's a good idea to celebrate your progress every month or so instead of waiting until you achieve your final goal, which could take a while. Taking pleasure in my small successes makes growing healthy a better experience than when I was constantly dieting and putting myself down!"

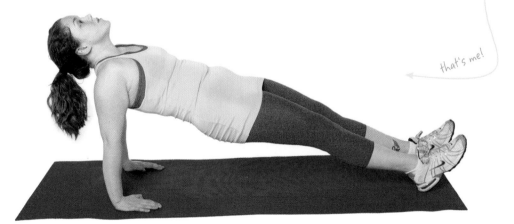

that's me!

147

Seriously, I HATE exercise.

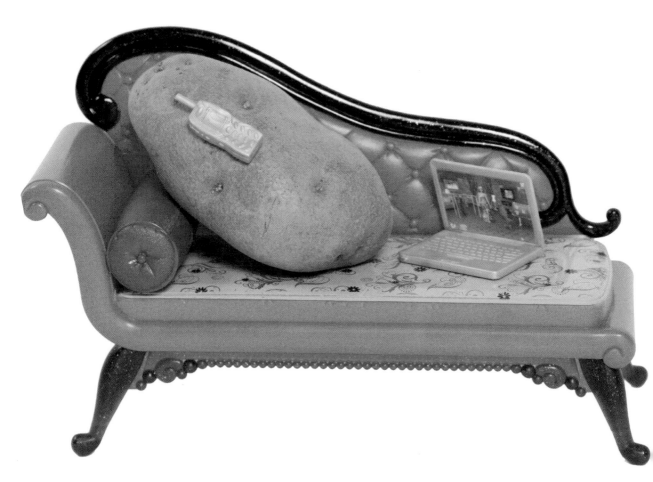

148

WHAT'S GOING ON?

Does the idea of breaking a sweat send shivers down your sofa-bound spine? Join the couch potato club that is the 70 percent of Americans who do no physical activity at all! Forty percent of inactive individuals say that the reason they don't move their bodies is that they don't enjoy exercise. But let's be honest: We do many things that we don't enjoy because we know they are good for us. So why make such a big deal about working out?

Common excuses from the exercise-is-evil club include:

There's nothing wrong with me. I don't need fixing. I'm fine as I am.

Life's too short and my time is too valuable to spend it cooped up in an overpriced, smelly gym.

I'd die if someone saw me in sweaty, stinky workout clothes.

It doesn't work. I tried once and didn't see any results.

I just don't want to, OK?

And many, many more reasons, all of which are addressed somewhere in this chapter already. Sadly, something that should be natural and routine, and even fun, has turned into a dreaded chore for many of us.

The problem is so prevalent that some researchers have defined a disorder called "exercise resistance." Whether on purpose or subconsciously (which means not thinking about their decision), exercise-resistant people sabotage their health because they don't move around enough to keep their bodies working well. Although not yet categorized as a mainstream disorder on par with anorexia or bulimia, exercise resistance starts from the same place. It is an expression of control over body and feelings. Just as you can't convince a girl with anorexia to "just eat a sandwich"—she'll come up with every excuse under the sun to avoid eating or simply ignore you and walk away—you can't tell an exercise-resistant person to stop being lazy and work out. Your advice will fall on deaf ears. And to make matters worse, exercise-resistant people are often binge eaters or compulsive overeaters, too. (See page 184 for more on eating disorders.)

HOW DO I DEAL?

Luckily, most of us aren't "exercise resistant"; we just aren't keen on the idea of going to the gym. And that's one of the biggest problems; we think exercise has to be done in a formal setting with fancy machines. But, as this chapter has demonstrated, that notion is all wrong! Many people who claim to hate exercise haven't given activity—or themselves—a fair chance, which is why it's so important to try these three steps before you give up on getting fit:

☆ Step 1) Find an activity you enjoy. Some people love the energy they get from working out with other exercisers at the gym or in group classes, while other people prefer exercising in their own private place. Don't throw in the towel until you've tried everything, and trying everything could take a few years. You can't use "there's nothing left to try" as an excuse to give up! The exercises in this book alone should keep you entertained for a few months. Also, try making slight changes to a workout routine that "almost works." Try listening to upbeat music, changing the type of clothing you wear, or exercising at a different time of day.

☆ Step 2) Grow up a little. I know firsthand that getting fit can be tough, especially when you don't like working out. That's why I've shared my personal stories about discovering new forms of exercise that I enjoy and can do often, such as triking and yoga. I want you to see that moving your body is not just possible, it's important. Be mature about the situation: Your health depends on it, so add your seven hours a week of working out to your calendar. It's as nonnegotiable as your bathroom breaks!

☆ Step 3) Give it time. You can't expect to love a new workout routine the first time you try it. Maybe not even the fifth time or the tenth time! I wasn't good at yoga at first, but I improved and I learned to enjoy it over time. Stay positive and remind yourself on rough days that you can look forward to improving not just the way your body looks but also the way you feel. You will grow stronger by the day, and your soreness will go away. Soon, exercise won't be "exercise." It will merely be a part of your daily routine—perhaps eventually the part that you look forward to the most!

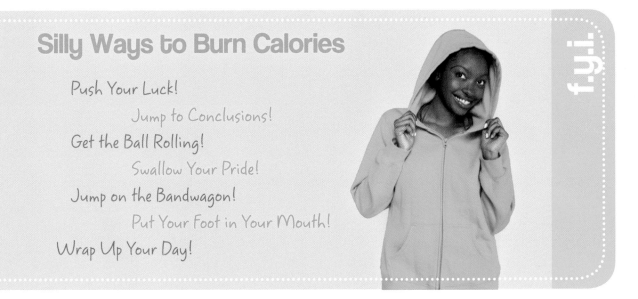

Silly Ways to Burn Calories

Push Your Luck!

Jump to Conclusions!

Get the Ball Rolling!

Swallow Your Pride!

Jump on the Bandwagon!

Put Your Foot in Your Mouth!

Wrap Up Your Day!

f.y.i.

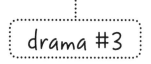

drama #3

I feel awful after I exercise.

WHAT'S GOING ON?

Exercise is supposed to energize your body, not drain your batteries! When you don't know how to pay attention to your body's warning signs and use common sense and tools such as the "Talk Test," exercising improperly or overexercising can make you feel weary and wary of working out again. Does your body throb from pushing yourself too hard and too fast? Are your toes raw from too-tight tennis shoes? Do you get dizzy because you skipped breakfast or didn't eat before you exercised?

These problems and others like them can make exercise downright painful, but you can easily avoid these mistakes and walk away from your workout feeling wonderful.

HOW DO I DEAL?

First, go back to page 92–93 and make sure that you're up to speed on exercise safety and that you've chosen the right sports bra. Next, from your toes to your head, check for problems that could be wrecking your routine:

✩ Shoes. Are you wearing the right kind of shoes when you exercise? Athletic shoes are different from cute sneakers. They have padding and protection to keep your feet and ankles safe and supported. A good pair can be purchased for $50 or less (especially if you find a sale), so put a new pair on your shopping list to purchase as soon as your wallet recovers from buying two sports bras. When shopping for shoes, always try them on at the end of the day, when your feet are at their largest, and don't buy them unless the shoes are already comfy to begin with. Athletic shoes shouldn't need "breaking in." For general exercise, buy shoes labeled for running or cross-training, but you may want sport-specific shoes if you have a favorite activity such as soccer or basketball. Make sure your shoes aren't too loose or tight. If your feet are narrow, wide, or two different sizes (more common than you may think!), consider shoes that have more than one set of eyelets so you can adjust your laces accordingly.

✩ Clothes. Do your workout clothes fit well? Too tight and your circulation is cut off, making you feel sick; too loose and you may be dealing with body burns and chafing from the friction (see page 156 for more).

✩ Water and food. Have you eaten and drunk enough water? Dehydration (too little water in your body) and hunger will make you feel weak and tired during and after your workout. Make sure that you've eaten something light but nutritious,

fast fact

Shoes or socks? If you're sure your shoes fit properly, check your socks. If they're threadbare or thin, they might not provide the cushioning you need. Buying five pairs of high-quality exercise socks (often $8-$12 a pair) can save you hundreds of dollars in blister pads and foot cream!

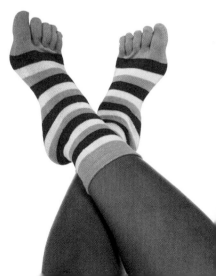

such as a handful of nuts or toast with peanut butter, about a half-hour before you exercise. And don't forget to take your water bottle with you!

☆ Intensity level. Are you going as hard and as fast as you can? Working hard may earn you an A+ for effort, but if you're overdoing it, you'll fail your body. Don't "push through" pain. Pain is your body's way of telling you to slow down. While it's important to break a sweat, there's no need to sweat buckets. When you're in your target intensity range (when you can carry on a conversation with some effort) you're achieving your health and body goals better than if you're wheezing and feeling ready to fall over.

Finally, it's normal to feel a little sore the day after a tough workout, but if you suffer from joint or knee pain, you may be doing something wrong or you may be injured. If you feel any kind of pain, talk to a professional trainer or healthcare provider before you move forward. You may need a brace or athletic tape for support while you're getting fit, or you may need to take things easy for a while to let an injury heal.

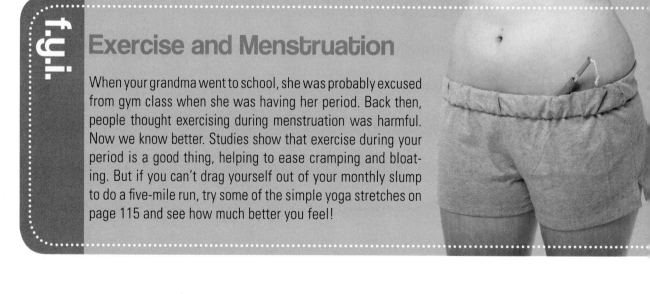

f.y.i.

Exercise and Menstruation

When your grandma went to school, she was probably excused from gym class when she was having her period. Back then, people thought exercising during menstruation was harmful. Now we know better. Studies show that exercise during your period is a good thing, helping to ease cramping and bloating. But if you can't drag yourself out of your monthly slump to do a five-mile run, try some of the simple yoga stretches on page 115 and see how much better you feel!

Rest Your Body!

Now that you're making time to move your body, make sure you set aside enough time for sleep. It's not a waste of time. In fact, sleep will help you achieve your slimming goals, while being sleep-deprived might just make you gain weight! In one study, researchers found that people who sleep six hours each night are more likely to be obese than those who sleep eight or nine hours. The risk of obesity increased by 30 percent for every hour of TV watching and decreased by 24 percent for every hour of sleeping! Does this mean you have to sleep your life away? No way! After studying one thousand people, researchers found that only twenty extra minutes of sleep per night was associated with a lower, healthier body weight, so hit the hay a half-hour earlier than usual and see if it helps!

Even if you don't want to slim down, your brain and body need plenty of sleep. Nine hours a night is recommended for teenagers, and those who sleep that long have higher grades, healthier bodies, and happier attitudes. If you go to school, work a job, play sports, and participate in many activities, getting nine hours a night may be a challenge, but you'll gain a lot from increasing your snooze time. If all else fails, stop staying up so late on the weekends and try catching up on some of the sleep you've missed during the week! Notice how much better you feel. Prioritizing your health by moving and resting more will enable you to better enjoy your remaining free time.

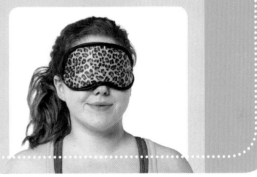

BTW: POWER NAPS ARE NICE

Never underestimate the power of a short snooze. It's important to strive for those nine hours a night, but if you're not getting that much, then try enjoying a fifteen- to twenty-minute siesta during the day (after school, perhaps) to give your brain a break. Many studies show that nappers learn better, perform better in sports, and enjoy better health than their non-napping peers!

Chafing

When you're exercising, do ever you feel as if your thighs might start a forest fire or your nipples might bleed? If you do, you're chafing, which simply means that your body parts are rubbing against something, either another body part or your clothes. When you sweat, chafing can grow worse. While the two most common areas for chafing are between your thighs and on your nipples, chafing can happen anywhere on the body! A snug waistband, a tight pair of panties, or a wrinkly sock can do damage, too. Blisters on your feet are a form of chafing. Once, after a long walk on a hot day, I realized that the underwire in my bra had been rubbing like sandpaper underneath my breasts, causing dark, painful lines that didn't disappear for days. And don't get me started on thong burn!

It's difficult to stick to a workout plan when chafing is cramping your style, so prevent it by:

☆ **Stopping sweat.** Use powder to keep chafe sites dry and sliding safely. Almost all body powders (including cornstarch, which is cheap) work well, but beware of fragrances and chemicals near sensitive spots. Test new products beforehand and read the list of ingredients on the label. You don't want to end up with a menthol burn in place of a chafe. Try making your own body powder with the recipe on page 158.

☆ **Freezing friction.** Banish friction by applying an anti-chafing powder or a thin coat of petroleum jelly to the problem areas. If that's not strong enough, check out your drugstore, where you'll find a variety of chafe prevention products. Beware that greasy stains from some products are nearly impossible to get out of clothes, so don't use those products if you're exercising in your favorite outfit.

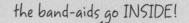

the band-aids go INSIDE!

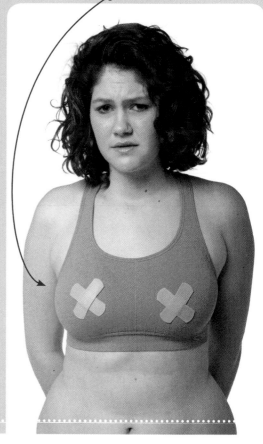

☆ **Protecting body parts.** Nipple guards are available to protect your girls, but if you're on a budget or can't find them, carefully placed Band-Aids can do the trick. Remember to remove them slowly and preferably in the shower to avoid an OUCH moment!

☆ **Choosing chafe-proof clothes.** Take a lesson from Goldilocks when you shop for workout clothes; not too tight and not too loose but JUST RIGHT! Choose natural fabrics such as cotton; synthetics trap sweat and moisture, making chafing worse. Keep your thighs from rubbing together by wearing body-hugging bike shorts or leggings. If your panties are the culprit, try going commando (no panties) or wear boy-cut underwear to minimize contact with body folds. At the first sign of chafing, remove any item that may be causing you discomfort. The more you sweat and move, the worse the chafing will get.

If your body has already been burned—literally—try these tips:

☆ **Get out of the awful attire.** Get your clothes off, take a shower, and hang out in your bedroom butt-naked for a while. Give your body a chance to cool off, calm down, and heal before subjecting it to clothes and motion again.

☆ **Get clean.** Grime and gunk can make chafing worse. It can even cause an infection. Wash yourself with mild soap and make sure you rinse well so you don't leave any soap on the irritated skin.

☆ **Get dry.** Towel off gently until there's no more moisture. Don't miss belly rolls, breast folds, underarms, your butt crack, and any place else where a crease can cause more chafing.

☆ **Treat the target spots.** If your skin is not broken, use gentle powders and petroleum jelly to soothe the soreness. If the burn is severe or the area seems inflamed, use a hydrocortisone cream or zinc oxide from the drugstore to tame the pain. If your skin cracks, oozes pus, or bleeds, see a doctor.

☆ **Watch out.** If the chafe doesn't go away in a few days—especially in the crotch area—call your doctor! You could have an infection that can be treated with over-the-counter medicine, but you must be properly diagnosed before beginning treatment.

HOW TO Make Your Own Anti-Chafing Powder

Are you worried about what might be in your store-bought powders and creams, or are you hoping to save some money? Here's an easy-to-make powder that can go in your pits, between your legs, at the nape of your neck, or wherever you need to feel fresh, dry, and chafe-free.

WHAT YOU'LL NEED:
a tablespoon, baking soda, cornstarch, and a clean resealable container

DIRECTIONS
Step 1) Dump 2 tablespoons of baking soda into the container. Add 12 tablespoons of cornstarch.
Step 2) Close the lid of the container and shake hard for about a minute to make sure the ingredients mix.
Step 3) Dab away. You can use a cosmetics puff or a cotton ball if you'd like, or your hands will do. You can also poke holes in some plastic containers to make sprinkle bottles if you want!

BTW: SMELLING BAD

To mask sweat odors, always apply an antiperspirant deodorant to clean pits before you exercise. If that doesn't stop the reek, think about what you chow down on. The odors of some foods and spices, such as garlic and onions, can make their way out of your body through your sweat. Try limiting those stinky seasonings and see if you notice a difference. Finally, if you're still smelly when working out despite your efforts, hold your head high. Sweat and odor mean that your body is burning calories and building strength, and you should feel proud knowing that you're working to improve yourself! And unless someone sniffs your pits or your crotch before you shower, chances are that the only person who can smell you is you!

I can't exercise enough
to burn off all the calories I eat.

WHAT'S GOING ON?

I certainly hope not! The point of exercise is not to burn off all the calories you eat in a day. Remember the information on metabolism on page 89? Your body burns a base number of calories just keeping you alive and moving. So if you are an active girl who needs 1,800 calories a day just to sustain these basic functions, the idea is NOT to burn that many with calories with exercise. You would have to jog for four hours nonstop to make that happen! If

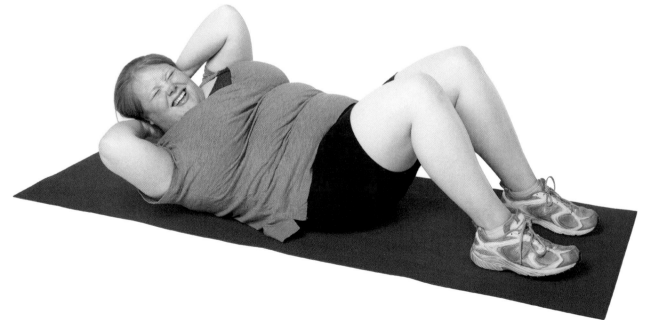

fast fact

Do you live in a dangerous neighborhood or cold climate where you can't exercise outside? Do you live in an unhappy home where working out is the last thing you want to (or can) do? If the answer is yes, try some other places such as your school gym or an after-school program. Many community centers have gymnasiums and exercise equipment you can use; all you have to do is ask!

belly laughs

What runs but never gets tired?

Water!

you're thinking, "I would never eat 1,800 calories in a day," then turn to page 166 to start reading about the importance of eating enough to fuel your body.

If you're thinking, "I've got to jog for four hours, then," you may be one of thousands of young women who are addicted to exercise. Now don't go calling Aerobics Anonymous just yet. Exercise addiction, also known as compulsive exercise, is real, but rare. Many who suffer from it don't realize they have a problem. You should seek help from a trusted adult if you:

- exercise despite pain and injury
- are obsessed with burning as many calories as possible
- are disappointed in your performance no matter how hard you push
- get jittery if you don't work out
- never give yourself a rest day

Compulsive exercisers go beyond loving the way working out makes them feel; they fret and obsess over gaining weight or losing muscle tone to the point where working out is all they think about. Compulsive exercisers are always pushing themselves to do more and go for longer, and overexercising is often coupled with an eating disorder such as anorexia or bulimia (more on page 184). Exercise addicts often exercise late at night so no one knows they are doing extra stomach crunches, leg lifts, or push-ups. They walk or run for miles every day in addition to visiting the gym, even if they're in pain. These extremes point to the problem called exercise addiction.

HOW DO I DEAL?

First, know that if you're a teen girl who is exercising for an hour a day and eating a healthy 1,600-2,000 calories every day, you're going to have no problem staying the same weight or slimming down. You'll learn more about food and calories in the next chapter, but you don't need to take exercise and eating healthily to extremes to see results!

Next, if you see yourself in one or more of the warning signs of exercise addiction, you may need to back off and evaluate why you're exercising so much. The point of exercise is to get your body in shape healthily, and there *is* such a thing as too much, unhealthy exercise. Especially if you've been pushing through pain or an injury, see your doctor to make sure you haven't done damage to your body. Ask a physician or counselor to help you get a handle on the emotions that are prompting you to exercise too much.

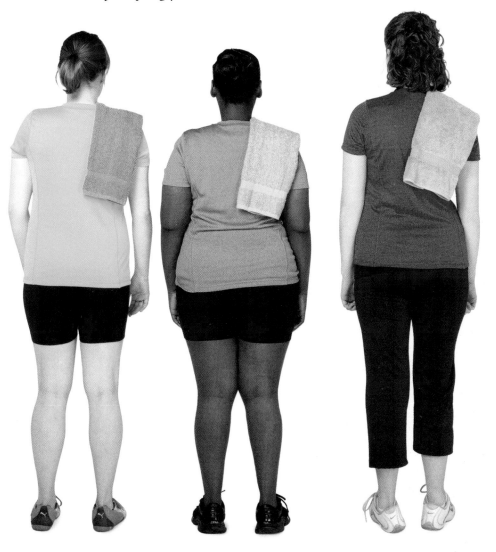

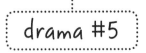

drama #5

I don't have the time to exercise.

WHAT'S GOING ON?

If your favorite celebrity called you up and said, "Meet me at the gym in fifteen minutes," you'd find a way, ANY WAY, to get there, right? Or how about if a game show called and said, "If you can run a mile in ten minutes, we'll give you a million dollars." You'd find a way to rearrange your calendar to start training, even if it meant running in place in your closet, wouldn't you? While the motivations for working out aren't usually that exciting, here's the point: If exercise matters to you, you can make time. Time is all about your mind-set!

If you make time for exercise now, you'll reap the benefits later. Who knows when you'll need to run to catch up with a cute person or heft fifteen dresses to the cash register at an all-you-can-carry-for-one-price clothing sale? Exercising now also means that come prom or summertime, you won't be tempted to dive into some stupid crash diet that doesn't work. You'll already be in the best shape of your life!

HOW DO I DEAL?

Take an honest look at how you spend your time before saying there's none left for exercise. TV, computers, movies—you and I both know that you can trim a few minutes off those extra activities to make room for an hour of activity each day, or at least something close to it. When you're bored, try doing something active instead of surfing channels or the Internet. Or, if you MUST see your favorite shows, incorporate your exercise into your viewing: You can always do strength training or yoga while watching your soaps!

If you truly believe you have no free time for exercise, not even twenty minutes a day, try using the tips on page 101 to increase the intensity of your daily activities. And take a look at the next "HOW TO" for ways to squeeze some exercise into your super-busy schedule.

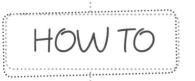

HOW TO Squeeze Exercise into Your Schedule

Thinking you don't have time is not an option. You must MAKE time to move your body. How? First, what's your average day really like? Track your hour-by-hour schedule to see where you can squeeze in some time for exercise, and separate the mandatory things (meaning you have to do them) from the optional activities.

In your twenty-four-hour day:

☆ How much time do you spend sleeping? (Hopefully at least 8-9 hours a day.) _____

☆ How much time do you spend at school or doing homework? (Probably 8-10 hours a day.) _____

☆ How much time do you spend eating, showering, and getting dressed? (Maybe 1-3 hours a day.) _____

☆ How much time do you spend at an after-school job or doing community service? _____

☆ Total the mandatory hours: _____

☆ Subtract this number from 24: 24 − _____ = _____

Well lookie-here. There seems to be some time left over, right? For nearly all of us, the time spent on mandatory activities adds up to somewhere between sixteen and twenty-two hours. That leaves two hours or more for squeezing in some exercise. And that's not counting weekends, holidays, and summers!

If your day includes two or three hours of computer fun, telephone talk, and TV watching, then rethink how busy you are and make the time to take care of yourself. If getting healthy matters to you, which it should, you may have to face some hard facts and cut back on the lounging to get in some lunging!

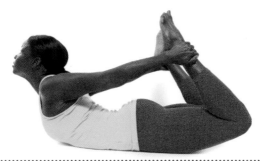

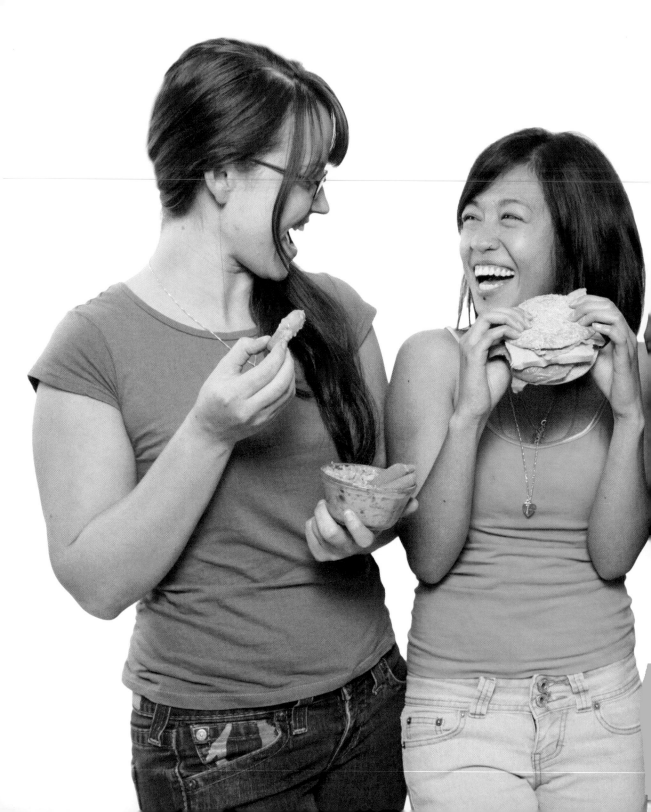

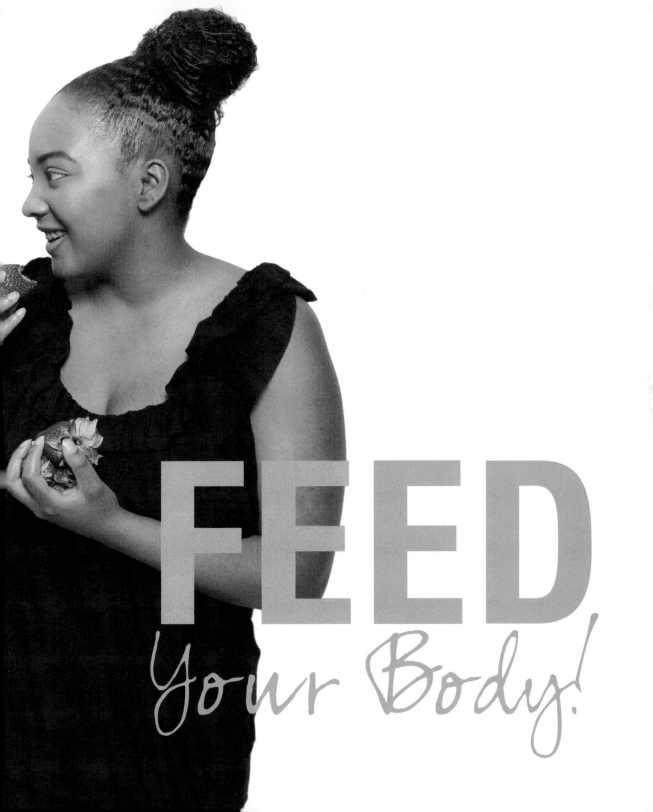

FEED *Your Body!*

I once joined a volunteer program at my high school just for the hot boys during and the hot food after. Yummy from start to finish! Once a week, after working up an appetite helping my community, I'd get in line for humongous helpings (at least two) of mouth-watering macaroni-and-cheese, blissful barbecue sandwiches, and coconut cake that I still crave. Back then I had total confidence in my body just as it was, and I happily gorged myself the day before I left to compete in my first beauty pageant. When I returned home without the title, blaming my body for my defeat, I started to try to lose weight, but I didn't stop volunteering. (Crushes are a calorie-free pleasure.)

Before my next community service event, I checked the calorie counts of some of my favorite foods served there, and the sky-high numbers encouraged me to get some control over the size of my portions. When it came time to chow down and my mentor noticed my plate heaping with salad but holding only a few spoonfuls of her specialties, she cried, "Girl, I made the macaroni extra cheesy just for you, and you're not eating any?"

I was embarrassed, but my personal goals did not involve a half pound of Velveeta. "I'm sorry. I just want to get in shape

We usually don't know what foods are good for us, and we

before going to college," I replied sweetly, hoping my words would win her over.

"Suit yourself," she answered, "but why are you avoiding the veggies? These green beans are good for you." That had been true when the beans were fresh-picked from her garden. However, by the time they made it to the back of her minivan, those beans had been boiled until few nutrients were left, fried in grease, mixed with bacon, and heavily salted. Sure, they tasted delicious, like OMG delicious, but calling them health food was false!

My dear mentor, who wanted nothing but the best for me, had no idea that her words were untrue. Although she was a hometown hero who changed many of her students' lives, when it came to influencing food choices, sharing nutrition facts, and demonstrating proper portion sizes, she was a community criminal!

It's easy to fool ourselves into believing that we're eating right. We usually don't know what's good for us, and we mistakenly believe that most healthy foods don't taste good. After reading this chapter, you'll be armed with the information you need to make the right food choices for your health. You'll learn how to eat not just for fun but to feel satisfied, and you'll find out how to cut out emotional eating and that always unnecessary third piece of cake!

mistakenly believe that most healthy foods don't taste good!

WHAT DOES IT MEAN TO FEED My Body?

By definition, food is anything solid or liquid that is taken into the body to sustain life, provide energy, and promote growth. But in practice, feeding your body is about more than eating to survive. How we feed our bodies says a lot about how much we value ourselves, what we know about food, and what is going on in our lives. Feeding your body the right way means that you have a healthy relationship with food. You know your body's food needs, you do your best to balance your plate, and you care about the quality of the food you consume. Sounds simple, right? Technically, it is, but in real life, it's tough to achieve those goals!

A whopping 95 percent of teen girls don't eat nearly the recommended amount of fruits and vegetables, and 91 percent don't get enough calcium from food to build strong bones and healthy bodies! Teen girls also aren't getting nearly enough of the fiber, water, vitamins, and minerals needed to grow and feel good. What we are getting more than enough of, however, is the things that no one needs in any great quantity: salt, sugar, fat, and chemicals from unhealthy processed foods. Processed foods have been altered or pre-cooked to be more convenient, quick-cooking, or tasty. Such foods contain a lot of calories, but they have little nutritional value (more on processed foods on page 206).

It's possible to eat nothing but junk and maintain a normal weight (especially if you move your body a lot), but while you may not increase your size, you might be decreasing your life span! Unhealthy eating habits kill more people than alcohol, drugs, and car accidents combined! Even if you don't suffer death by donuts in the long run, eating badly can have some serious and unappealing consequences in the short run. Eating badly can make you feel tired, moody, bloated, slow, lazy, unintelligent, and depressed. What you choose to consume affects everything about your body—your skin, hair, nails, teeth, even your poop!

If your eating habits are bad but you're reading this thinking, "But I feel okay," you probably have no idea how good you can feel when you feed your body with healthy foods! You might not know what life is like without battling acne, craving caffeine, or unbuttoning tight pants because your stomach feels bloated after a chemical-filled junk food meal. Imagine not having to hit snooze every five minutes in the morning because you slept terribly! Imagine going to the bathroom without straining or pushing. (It's awesome!)

Although some of us with certain body types will be always bigger, even if we do eat healthily and exercise, no one needs to suffer from health problems and illnesses brought on by drinking too many milk shakes and eating too much mayonnaise. I know from personal experience, however, that eating better is not as easy as simply cutting out the foods that aren't good for us. Why? Because food is often tied to feelings. When you want to treat yourself, don't you often ask for your favorite food to make the fun complete? Does food help soothe you when you feel sad or depressed? Comfort foods are a normal part of life: We expect chicken soup when we're sick and cake when we're celebrating. But many of us unknowingly develop an unhealthy relationship with food; we become emotionally attached to food and—lacking knowledge of nutrition and someone to encourage us to eat better—we continue in our comfortable eating patterns that become harder and harder to break free from.

Because processed foods are so cheap and easy to obtain, more and more of us now refuse to eat much of anything that's not frozen or junk food. (I recently met a girl who won't eat anything except chicken nuggets for dinner, lunch, AND breakfast.) But even when we are actually trying our best to eat better (70 percent of teen girls say they want to improve their eating habits), the effort is extremely difficult because we aren't armed with the right information or the fridge full of healthy foods that we need to start feeding our bodies the right way!

While it is recommended that schools should teach about food and nutrition for fifty hours each year, the average student only receives three to six hours of nutritional education annually, leaving behind many more questions than answers. Are carbs the enemy? Or is it fat? If sugar is so bad, what's wrong with living on artificial sweeteners? Why didn't anyone tell us that a salad drenched in blue cheese dressing isn't healthier—or even lower in calories—than a cheeseburger? Or that there are no bad foods, only bad portion sizes? (Okay, I admit there *are* a *few* bad food ingredients; see page 216 for the short list.) And what about the fact that skipping meals causes weight *gain*?

When we don't have the facts, we often end up making the wrong food choices. We give up and order the chicken tenders combo with onion rings and a large soda because it's easy, cheap (sorta, see page 238 for why it's not really), filling, and socially acceptable because it's what our friends are eating. Best of all, the food is delicious, especially when super-salty, fried flavor is all we know.

Beginning today and using the information in this chapter, stop letting what you eat control you and your feelings. Instead, start seeing what food can do for you!

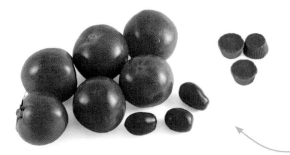

Three tiny, unhealthy-fat filled caramel cups have the same number of calories as more than six delicious, healthy, and filling tomatoes! Turn to page 202 for more visuals.

WHY SHOULD I
FEED My Body?
Instead of Going on a Diet?

Because DIETS DON'T WORK! Not only is the word *diet* loaded with painful associations, the act of dieting has been proven to *promote* weight *gain*! The definition of a diet is a limitation on food consumed for the purpose of losing weight. We already know that food is tied to our feelings, and when dieters feel that something they are emotionally attached to (food) is being taken away, resentment and rebellion take over! Most of us fail when we diet because we consider dieting a punishment or a chore, and as with all chores or punishments, we ALWAYS try to cut corners and/or do things sloppily to get them over with. While no one gets hurt if you hastily use your brother's towel to mop the bathroom floor (and then put it back on the rack where it was, hee hee), when you starve yourself or use stupid supplements to slim down faster, someone does get hurt, and that someone is YOU. Since weight loss occurs when we burn more calories than we consume, it's easy for us to think that eating as few calories as possible should speed up the process. But as you'll learn starting on page 174, the way our bodies work involves more than simple math!

The recommended number of calories you need to eat to stay healthy (page 178) probably seems a lot higher than what you're used to in a diet plan (page 180 explains why). If you are trying to lose weight, the scale might not show weight loss as fast as you'd like—but remember that you shouldn't be hopping on the scale all the time anyway. Studies show that people who shape up slowly through exercise and eating healthily stay slimmer for longer than those who go on starvation diets. Always eating properly and exercising will help you look great not just after a crash diet but for the rest of your life! So stop dragging your body through one damaging diet after another and turn the page to begin the journey toward a healthier, happier relationship with food!

Wacky Diets THROUGH HISTORY

1900-1910 – The Chew-Chew Diet. The dieter could eat anything she wanted, but the rule was that every bite had to be chewed thirty-two times before tilting the head back and sliding the sludge down the throat. Before you say, "That's not too hard," try it. It's torture.

1910-20s – Tapeworms. Although no remaining samples of tapeworm-containing pills are still around today, these nutrient-sucking critters were rumored to be the cause of a few celebrities' successes in slimming, starting at the turn of the twentieth century. I've read gross tales about how, after the diet worked its "magic," the dieter faced the trauma of expelling the worm through the mouth by enticing it with a glass of warm milk. Ew!

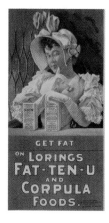

1930s-50s – Weight Gain Tablets. Slim wasn't always in style, so instead of starving themselves, many women spent their savings on mail-order products that promised to help them gain the weight they needed to be fashionable. One ad announced that "skinny girls are not glamour girls" and urged women ashamed of a "skinny, scrawny figure" to buy a vitamin formula to "help you add pounds and pounds of firm, attractive flesh to your figure."

1920s-40s – Smoking. Even today, teen girls who are trying to lose weight are more likely to start smoking than those who are not, but at least we aren't subjected to ads suggesting that smoking is normal and healthy. In 1928, one brand went as far as to say, "To keep a slender figure, no one can deny, reach for a cigarette instead of a sweet." Women who followed that advice may have lost a few inches (probably not), but they also lost years off their lives!

1950s-Present – The Master Cleanse. Only a superstar like Beyoncé could convince millions of people worldwide (myself included) to stock up on lemons, cayenne pepper, maple syrup, and laxative tea in an effort to lose weight. But that's exactly what happened when she claimed to have lost twenty-two pounds in two weeks on the "Master Cleanse" diet, also known as the "Lemonade Diet." Many grocery stores reported selling out of lemons for months on end after Beyoncé told her story on *The Oprah Winfrey Show* in 2006. Beyoncé's "detox" has been around since the 1950s and it does the trick, making you temporarily thinner, but so would almost anything so restrictive. It works by dehydrating you—so much of what you lose is water weight and it causes not only the breakdown of excess fat, but also of muscle and lean body mass, which is the good stuff. And speaking from personal experience (I lasted three days and was so hungry afterward that I ended up gaining weight from my gorging), it is a miserable diet that only someone who is waited on hand and foot (like a multimillionaire celebrity) could truly complete without landing in jail for assaulting someone for a sandwich.

1960s – Relax-A-Cizor. Over 400,000 of these electric shock machines were sold up until 1970, when a federal judge declared them dangerous and ordered them off the market. These "passive exercise" devices were said to work by sending pulses of electrical charge through the body to contract muscles without effort. In truth, the machines caused miscarriages and worsened medical conditions including hernias, ulcers, and varicose veins.

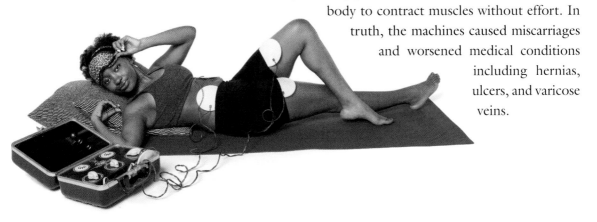

1975-present – The Cookie Diet. I don't know anyone who has lost weight on this, but it's still going strong. Supposedly, the cookies you are supposed to eat on the diet promise to stop hunger. You eat nothing but the cookies and a small dinner all day, for a total of fewer than 1,000 calories. If you don't already know what's wrong with this picture, turn to page 180 for why eating too few calories is bad for your body. Calories aside, any diet that restricts you to a single food item—cookies especially—is not sustainable. Eating better is not about a set period of time; it's about building habits for a lifetime.

HOW CAN I FEED *My Body?*

Whether you're sleeping all day or training to run a marathon, your body needs a certain amount of food for survival. There is a bare minimum needed to keep you alive and the amount of food you need increases with greater activity. That's why marathon runners usually have to eat a whole lot more than the rest of us just to stay the same size; they burn many calories when they run all day long!

As I said in the previous chapter, food is the only way to get energy into your body. The amount of energy that a certain food item has to offer the body is measured in calories, and calories are what set food apart from a tin can or a piece of glass. Every food source, from a stalk of celery to a piece of chicken to processed fake cheese, contains calories and different food sources contain different amounts of caloric energy (also known as calorie counts).

Food also contains other important substances: vitamins, minerals, water, and fiber, all of which are *nutrients*. While calories enable your body to survive, nutrients enable your body to *thrive*. Eating too few calories will cause your body to quit working after a while, but even if you get enough energy to survive, eating mostly "empty calories" that don't contain the right amounts or kinds of vitamins and minerals can bring on an array of health problems, including fatigue, hair loss, even blindness!

However, the problem most of us have isn't that we're eating too *few* calories on a daily basis; it's that we're eating *too many*—far too many, in fact. When you eat more calories than your body burns, that unused energy is stored somewhere in your body, eventually becoming body fat. A few days of eating extra calories won't make much of a difference, at least not right away. That's because calories take a while to add up. Think of gaining weight as something like going to an arcade and winning a few tickets for each game. Two or three tickets might not get you anything cool, but if you save them up over a few visits, you can claim a not-so-lame prize.

That's how extra calories work, except that the "prize" you get for an extra 3,500 stored calories is a pound of body fat.

OK, so you had two pieces cake at your birthday party and tried a fried candy bar at the fair—that's life, right? An occasional treat won't hurt because it is probably worked off the next day, especially if you're active. However, many of us aren't just eating extra calories occasionally. Whether we know it or not (because we're not paying attention to calorie counts or we don't know how many calories we should eat), we're chowing down on too many calories every day for weeks and months on end! On average, teens today eat up to 230 calories more per day than teens ate twenty years ago. Most of that increase comes from huge portions of nonnutritious processed food and "empty calories," which are food that contain few nutrients except calories. To put 230 calories into perspective, it's about the difference between an order of six chicken nuggets plain compared with ten chicken nuggets with barbecue sauce. It's also the difference between a small and a large order of French fries! Tell the truth. When's the last time you asked for a small order of fries?

When we consume more calories than our bodies need, we gain weight. A pound of body fat equals 3,500 calories, so unless we burn off those extra calories, they are stored as excess body fat. For example, suppose you eat only 200 more calories per day more than your body needs. They may not seem like much, but over a year, that adds up to 73,000 extra calories, or more than twenty pounds of excess body fat!

Does this mean you have to swear off your favorite foods forever? Of course not. Even French fries can fit into a healthy meal plan! Feeding your body the right amounts and kinds of good food can be fun—and you don't have to go hungry or give up great taste. A lot goes into understanding food and nutrition, but feeding your body begins when you:

✩ Know how much food your body needs. Find out how many calories are healthy for your age, activity level, and body goals, as well as how often you should eat.

✩ Balance your plate. Figure out how much of each food group you should fit into each day's meals, as well as how to serve yourself smartly with proper portion sizes.

✩ Care about what you consume. Start reading food labels so that you know exactly what you're eating; and learn food lingo so you know which ingredients to look for and which ones to avoid.

You FEED Your Body When You...
KNOW HOW MUCH FOOD YOUR BODY NEEDS

If you're a teen girl who hardly ever exercises, you probably burn about 1,800 calories a day just to stay alive and do your everyday tasks (see page 178). So if you want to stay the same size, you should eat about 1,800 calories daily. (This goes back to the "calories in, calories out" equations on page 88.) However, if your goal is to slim down, you should cut back by about 200 calories a day to 1,600—but never any fewer than that (see page 180 for why). Ideally, if you also start to exercise for an hour every day, you'll burn another 150 to 400 calories (depending on the type of activity). (Make sure to work up a sweat when you can and use the "Talk Test" on page 137 to stay safe.) However, the more active you are, the more calories you need to eat, so make sure you understand what your caloric needs are before cutting back!

By decreasing your calories eaten and increasing your calories burned you create what is called a "calorie deficit." Your weight can change from day to day because of fluctuating levels of water and salt in your body, but the only way to get rid of excess body fat for good is by burning more calories than you consume by exercising and eating right.

If you consume 200 fewer calories per day every day for a week (that's 1,400 fewer calories total), and, that same week spend an hour per day exercising, burning an average of 300 calories an hour, (that's 2,100 more calories burned), you'll create a deficit of 3,500 calories. Since a pound of body fat equals 3,500 calories, this deficit leads to a pound of weight loss per week, which is a safe, healthy goal for teens.

While a single pound sounds like a puny amount, you have to realize that your weight isn't the only factor that matters. Consider these other important facts:

fast fact

Studies are starting to show that the chemicals and additives in junk foods have an addictive quality not unlike drugs and alcohol. Don't let your cravings control your life! Break the addiction!

✩ **You're building muscle.** As you learned in the previous chapter, the stronger you become, the more calories your body burns all day long.

✩ **Other signs are more dramatic.** Use some of the health measurements suggested on page 42 and you'll instantly start to see improvements!

✩ **You're still growing.** You can't eat fewer than 1,600 calories because your body needs nutrients to get you through puberty. Seriously, you can be a fifteen-year-old petite, curvy girl and unexpectedly shoot up several inches in six months. Growth spurts are funny like that, and you don't want to throw them off track by eating too little. See page 180 to learn more about why you shouldn't underfeed your body.

To estimate how many calories you should consume, let's figure out how many calories you're burning in an average day by quizzing your activity level!

HOW TO Determine Your Caloric Needs

Answer each of the following questions by choosing the option that sounds most like you in an average week. Be honest! Don't pretend you're running three marathons a week or use your goal activity level to up the number of calories you can eat right now. Once you start your super workout plan, you can adjust your quiz results, but for now be honest about where you are starting.

I fit in an hour of sweating through sports or other exercise:
A) One day per week or less.
B) Two to four days per week.
C) Five to seven days per week.

If I drive to the mall and there are no parking spots close to the entrance, I usually:
A) Circle around for as long as it takes to get a spot near the door.
B) Grudgingly park in the faraway spot.
C) Take whatever spot is available and walk briskly to the mall entrance.

Added up, I climb ____ flights of stairs per day:
A) None
B) Three or four
C) Five or more

I sit and watch TV or use the computer:
A) More than three hours per day
B) About two or three hours per day
C) An hour or less per day.

If the elevator's broken and won't be fixed for twenty minutes and I have to get to the sixth floor, I :
A) Go get a snack and come back in 20 minutes.
B) Start up the stairs but complain the entire way up, barely making it without collapsing.
C) Sprint up the stairs without a second thought.

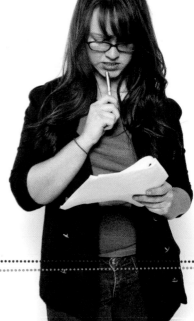

Mostly A's –You're **sedentary**, which is a fancy way of saying that your lifestyle leads you to move as little as possible. We may have to use a spatula to unstick you from your stubbornly seated position!

Mostly B's –You're **pretty active.** You could definitely make some lifestyle changes to get more movement in, but you're not a complete couch potato, so congrats!

Mostly C's –You're **very active**, which is great. Keep moving and shaking because no matter what your size is, you certainly can't be mistaken for a bump on a log or a slow-moving sloth!

What does your activity level have to do with what you eat? When you consider your activity level along with your age, you can figure out the right number of calories to consume.

TO STAY THE SAME SIZE

Age	Sedentary	Pretty Active	Very Active
14-18	1,800	2,000	2,400 calories per day

Now that you know how to stay the same size, the rest of the equation is easy! In order to burn off excess body fat, decrease your caloric intake by 200 calories per day.

TO SLIM DOWN

Age	Sedentary	Pretty Active	Very Active
14-18	1,600	1,800	2,200 calories per day

So, for safe weight loss, a sedentary sixteen-year-old might get by on 1,600 calories, but a very active sixteen-year-old might need around 2,200 calories to keep her body going on a busy day. Decreasing only 200 calories a day may not seem like a lot—it's equal to nine Hershey's Kisses—but when combined with additional physical activity, it packs a powerful punch. Be patient and you'll see results at a gradual but healthy rate.

No matter what, make sure you NEVER go below 1,600 calories a day without a doctor's advice (see page 180 for why)! If you're younger than fourteen, see your doctor for recommendations on how many calories are right for your body's needs.

ALWAYS EAT ENOUGH

I cannot stress this enough—no matter what, unless you're under doctor's orders, *you should NEVER eat fewer than 1,600 calories a day.* If you do, you run the risk of messing up your metabolism. One of the biggest mistakes that many of us make, aside from accidentally overeating in the first place, is assuming that cutting calories by more than 200 a day will speed up the process and cause us to slim down faster. It may, but the speedy weight loss will come at a high price! When you deprive your body of the minimum number of calories it needs to function normally, it will start hanging on tightly to the few calories you do give it, slowing your metabolism in an effort to survive. If you starve yourself for too long, eventually your body won't be able to readjust when you start eating normally again (which you will), and you will gain the weight back, and then some. Then, instead of being patient and waiting for your body to correct itself, you may try to cut calories even more, creating a cycle of starvation and damage.

You're probably used to seeing diets that scream smaller numbers of calories a day, but those aren't for you if you're a teen. If an adult female close to you has recently gone on a diet, you might have noticed that she ate fewer than 1,600 calories a day, even if she's the same height, weight, and activity level as you. The average teen girl burns calories faster than an adult does because her body is growing and changing. So, even when trying to slim down, you need more calories than most adults. Once your body stops growing in your late teens and early twenties, you will need less energy and your metabolism will slow. At that age you may find that you lose weight at 1,200-1,500 daily calories, but that amount is too low if you're younger than eighteen!

If you think you've already done some damage by dieting dangerously, don't spend the rest of your life worrying about whether your horrible habits are making your body refuse to lose; but don't keep trying the same tricks that don't work either! You can help your body heal, although the process may take time. Start eating a healthy amount of food today, and find a doctor or other health professional that you can talk to about food issues—past, present, and potentially in the future.

NEVER SKIP MEALS

Letting yourself get too hungry between meals increases the chance that you'll overeat when you do make time for a meal. Skipping meals also messes with your metabolism! But when you give your body small bursts of energy from food every few hours, you keep your body from shifting into "survival mode." When your body feels hungry too often, it starts holding onto calories and storing as many as possible in preparation for future starvation!

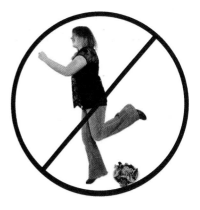

Too many of us have no idea how damaging it is to jump, hop, and skip right over meals. Over a third of girls ages thirteen to nineteen say they skip meals because they're busy, while 22 percent skip meals because they want to lose weight! Skipping meals won't help you lose weight. In fact, you may end up eating more: 21 percent of teen girls admit to binging after skipping meals. What's more, you're more likely to be an angry, confused mess when you don't eat enough. Your brain needs energy to work!

While we might not forget to put on our lip gloss in the morning, more than three out of five teen girls gloss over the most important meal of the day, breakfast. Whether in exchange

BTW: YOUR CALORIC NEEDS MAY VARY

While the calorie counts discussed here are a good guess, these numbers are not perfect because no two bodies are exactly alike. You may burn more calories as a sedentary person than a very active person your same age, perhaps because of your body composition or inherited traits. Or you may need fewer calories than suggested for those same reasons (but never fewer than 1600 per day). It's not unusual for athletes to need more than 3,000 calories a day to stay the same size. During competition time, twenty-five-year-old female Olympic weightlifter Carissa Gump chows down on 3,500 calories a day to stay at 139 pounds! If you notice that these recommendations aren't working for you after a month or two, see your doctor for specific suggestions on how many calories are right for you!

for an extra hour of sleep or a few calories saved, or just because we "don't feel hungry in the morning," many of us miss the morning meal. I was no stranger to skipping breakfast and hitting the snooze button myself, as revealed by my high school eating habits, which I share on page 183.

Not surprisingly, once I finally started eating breakfast, my body and my state of mind changed. Think about it: If you're supposed to eat every three or four hours, and you're sleeping for eight or nine, of course your body needs a jumpstart in the morning! Breakfast is also important because it helps you:

- ✿ think clearly
- ✿ get through the day without feeling tired
- ✿ do better on tests and schoolwork
- ✿ not binge on junk because you're ravenously hungry
- ✿ rev up your metabolism (see page 89), causing you to burn more calories all day long

Yes, it's true. Eating before your body tells you it needs to (with serious stomach growling and a bad attitude brewing) can cause you to burn more calories throughout the day.

Once you have breakfast down pat, don't skip lunch or dinner, either! And, your three main meals a day are important, but they're not all you need. For example, let's say that you are trying to slim down on 1,800 calories a day. If you limit yourself to three meals a day, each meal would be about 600 calories, which may be more food than you want at one time, especially if you're choosing healthy foods. But what if you're hungry in between? Smart snacking means that you never leave your body feeling super hungry. You can still eat 1,800 calories if you split them between three smaller meals and two snacks—it's better for you and you'll feel fuller! Turn to page 212 to learn how to read labels so that you can keep track of your calories and incorporate smart snacking in an easy and tasty way.

fast fact

Skipping breakfast is linked to excess body fat. Overweight teens are more likely to skip breakfast than their leaner friends.

I CONFESS:
I USED TO HAVE THE WORST EATING HABITS!

Oh, high school! How I remember not having the slightest idea how to feed my body. I'd skip breakfast to save time and pig out on a pile of French fries from the school cafeteria at lunch, washing everything down with an orange soda, which I mistakenly believed had nutritional benefits similar to orange juice. (It doesn't; see page 225 for other common food mistakes.) I'd get hungry an hour later and by the end of the school day, I would be ravenous and on edge, so before I'd hop on the bus (to be driven less than a mile to my house because I was too lazy to walk), I'd hit the snack machines for potato chips and another sugary soda to tide me over until I got home. On days when I had cheerleading practice, we'd always order fast food (and never the healthy options). One of my friends with a car would take our orders before practice began, pick up the food when it was over, and drop me off right after we had eaten more burgers, fries, and shakes than I care to think about. Then I would arrive home around dinnertime, but because I wasn't that hungry after the fast food, I'd skip the main courses Mom had made and go straight for the starches—picking the potatoes, trashing the tomatoes, breaking into the bread, and smothering my salad with mayonnaise-based ranch dressing, thinking that there was nothing wrong with my eating habits.

The first time I decided to "diet," the foods I ate changed a little, but not much else did. I still skipped breakfast, and I'd have only one item at lunch, usually a baked potato with a diet soda. I was pretty proud of myself. So few calories already! But, by the end of the day, I'd always be in a bad mood and hungry, so I'd usually "ruin" my diet by jumping right back into junk foods. Even when I ate what I thought was "better" for me, I'd serve myself too much. A huge plate heaped with pasta and tomato sauce is not one serving—it's six! And I'd add on extra calories that I didn't think about counting, such as dressings, cheese, and bacon bits on my salads. (See page 235 for better salad toppings.) By the time I read enough health information to realize that I wasn't eating often enough, or eating the right kinds or amounts of foods, I'd already wasted a couple of months, and the only thing I'd lost was sixty days!

Eager Dieter or Eating Disorder?

There's a fine line between dieting and an eating disorder, but millions overstep it every year. Nearly 6 percent of women and almost 3 percent of men have an eating disorder. That may not sound like many, but it's one out of every eleven adults you know, and the numbers may well be higher among teens!

People with eating disorders come in all shapes and sizes, from all ethnicities, religions, backgrounds, and financial situations. No group is exempt. You may not "look" as if you have an eating disorder, but you may have one all the same. Here is a short look at some common and not so common eating disorders:

✪ **Bulimia.** People with bulimia eat more food than they need to and then try to get rid of the extra calories by throwing up, using laxatives, fasting, or overexercising. Vomiting wreaks havoc on your teeth and breath, causes dry skin and chapped lips, and breaks blood vessels around the eyes (from the strain of vomiting). Abuse of laxatives causes tremors, weakness, blurry vision, fainting, kidney damage, and, in extreme cases, death. People with bulimia come in all shapes and sizes, from very small to extremely large.

✪ **Anorexia nervosa.** The word *anorexia* simply means "loss of appetite," but people with anorexia nervosa have an obsessive fear of eating and gaining weight. Their body image is distorted and they can starve themselves down to extremely low weights if they don't get treatment in time. Even as their bones start to protrude, the hair on their head falls out, and excess body hair starts to grow, people with anorexia frequently cannot overcome their fear of weight gain without professional help. While we commonly use the term *anorexic* to mean very thin, people with anorexia come in all shapes and sizes, too.

We hear a lot about anorexia and bulimia as mental health issues, but many more people binge eat and overeat. Their eating disorders are just as serious. Overeating and refusing to exercise are disorders that start with the mind, too.

✪ **Binge eating.** Binge eaters consume huge amounts of food in a single sitting, and the extra calories are stored as excess body fat. Sometimes, binge eaters skip meals and starve themselves, eating nothing for long periods of time before they binge, creating a cycle of unhealthy food habits and interfering with normal metabolism. Binge eaters can be all shapes and sizes, from very small to extremely large.

☆ **Compulsive overeating.** Compulsive overeaters rarely go long without eating. Eating is like a nervous tic or an obsession for them. In the same way people with anorexia can't "just start eating," overeaters can't "just stop"—not without professional help anyway. Compulsive overeating is common among extremely large individuals.

☆ **Exercise resistance.** Exercise-resistant people are also often binge eaters and/ or compulsive overeaters, refusing to move their bodies no matter how much sense it makes to do so. See page 149 for more.

If you feel that you are mentally or physically unable to take care of yourself and feed your body, or even if you're not sure, know that you are not alone. Talk to your doctor about your concerns and check out some resources and health Web sites (page 242) to get back on track when it comes to treating your body right.

DIET Pills

f.y.i.

I talk about diet pills in *Body Drama* on page 223, and I can't stress this point enough: DON'T USE THEM. Here's the short version of why not:

☆ **They're addicting.** Becoming addicted to diet pills is common, even when the pills don't work. And downing diet pills can be the gateway to other dangerous disorders.

☆ **They're dangerous (duh).** Just because it's for sale doesn't mean that it's safe. When diet pills first became popular in the 1930s, they killed some users and blinded others. Times haven't changed much. Many people are injured or killed by over-the-counter weight-loss products each year.

☆ **They don't work.** Diet pills are temporary fixes, if any fix at all; but worse, they leave behind permanent problems with your metabolism, heart function, and more. Fourteen percent of teen girls have tried dangerous diet pills to lose weight. While that might sound scary, remember: 86 percent of girls are doing things the right way (meaning no diet pills at all)! STEER CLEAR of diet pills and shape up the right way!

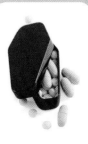

You FEED Your Body When You...
BALANCE YOUR PLATE

Have you ever wished that a balanced diet meant having a cookie in both hands? Counting calories can be a bit of a chore, and you can't always know the calorie counts of what you're eating, such as your neighbor's amazing sweet potato soufflé. Still, you can make sure that you're feeding your body well if you fit in all of the food groups and serve yourself portions of the proper size.

Balancing your plate can be difficult at first, but it becomes easier with practice. Luckily, perfection isn't the goal. You don't have to count every peanut to know that a small handful is one serving. And you don't have to carry around the Queen of Hearts to know that a proper

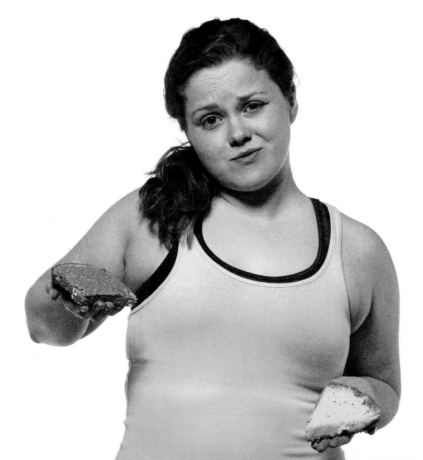

portion of meat is about the size of a deck of cards. Balancing your plate is about common sense. It helps you remember to eat food from all the food groups, and it lets you judge how much of a food is too much!

FIT IN ALL THE FOOD GROUPS

Living off of leftover Halloween candy for a couple of days isn't going to ruin your health, but in the long run you need to eat a wide variety of foods to get all the energy and the different types of nutrients you need to stay healthy.

Without the right amounts of energy and nutrients we:

- ✩ tire more easily
- ✩ get sick more often
- ✩ don't grow as strong as we might
- ✩ feel moody and depressed

Everything edible contains nutrients, but some foods are lacking in the nutrition department while others are packed with the good stuff. To help us make the right choices, foods that contain similar types and amounts of nutrients are categorized in six main groups: vegetables, dairy, fruits, grains, protein, and fats.

Some people who are trying to slim down cut out grains or fats, thinking that these are the culprits in their weight gain. Unless you're allergic (see page 195), this approach is not smart! While some grains and fats are better than others, eliminating the good kinds with the bad hurts you and your health. Instead of giving up certain kinds of foods altogether, choose foods from all the groups and avoid those that are low in nutritional value, such as added sugars and the "bad" fats: cholesterol, saturated fat, and trans fat (see page 223 for more).

fast fact

Eat the rainbow! Healthy foods come in a range of colors, and usually, the brighter and more diverse your meals are, the more nutrients you're consuming, so mix up your colors for a pretty plate!

fast fact

A food may be placed in a certain primary category, but it may also have nutrients that occur in another food group. For example, beans are protein foods, but they are actually fruits (although they are usually considered vegetables).

fast fact

Substituting pasta, beans, and soups for meat two or three times per week can save you $780 a year. Cutting out your afternoon trip to the vending machines for a soda and chips can save $500 or more. Think of the wonderful things you can do with all that cash!

Here are the daily food group guidelines for teen girls:

☆ Vegetables. 2–3 servings/cups per day, raw or steamed whenever possible to retain the most nutrients. 1 cup = one serving, so strive for 2–3 cups of veggies every day. 1 cup serving examples include 12 baby carrots, 10 broccoli florets, one large bell pepper, or one small ear of corn. 2 cups of salad greens counts as 1 serving.

☆ Grains. 6 servings/ounces per day, at least 3 of which should be whole grain, not refined (see page 208 to find out the difference). For grains, 1 ounce = 1 serving, and grains come in a variety of weights, so portion examples that are about 1 ounce each include 1 cup of breakfast cereal flakes; ½ cup of cooked oatmeal, rice, or pasta; 1 slice of bread; 5 whole wheat crackers; or ½ of an 8-inch tortilla.

☆ Protein. 2½–3 servings/5½–6 ounces per day, most of which should come from vegetable or lean meat sources and not battered and fried. For protein, 2–3 ounces = 1 serving. Proteins come in a variety of forms, so serving examples that are about 2–3 ounces each include 2 tablespoons of peanut butter (2 ounces) and 2 turkey sandwich slices (2 ounces). A piece of meat the size of a deck of cards counts as 2.5–3 ounces (more on eyeballing servings on page 196).

fast fact

Portions and servings aren't the same. A serving is a carefully measured recommended amount (see, for example, the serving sizes on nutrition labels, page 212). A portion is the amount of food actually consumed. Many times, a single portion, especially in restaurants and from packaged foods, contains multiple servings.

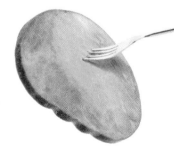

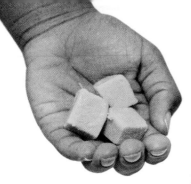

✩ Dairy. 3 servings/cups per day, sticking to lowfat cheese, milk, and yogurt to avoid saturated fat (page 223). With dairy, 1 cup = one serving. 1 cup portion examples include 1 individual yogurt container (8 oz.) and 1 half-pint container of milk. 1.5 oz. of cheese counts as 1 cup.

fast fact

Twelve baby carrots? A piece of chicken the size of a deck of cards? Half of a tortilla? Do these serving sizes sound super small to you? You are not alone! Turn to page 196 to learn more about how much you're really supposed to be putting on your plate.

✩ Fruits. 2 servings/cups per day, preferably not all as juice in order to obtain the most nutrition (even if you choose 100 percent juice). 1 cup serving examples include a fist-sized apple, 32 grapes, a cup of 100 percent fruit juice, or an 8-inch banana.

✩ Fats. 5 teaspoons per day of "added" fats—this is less than two tablespoons. The right kinds of fats are great for our health, and up to 30 percent of our calories need to come from them, but preferably from within other foods in other food groups (such as peanut butter or almonds or avocados). The fats to watch are those that we use as seasonings and spreads, such as mayonnaise, butter, and salad dressings; the large amounts of cooking oil used in preparing such foods as French fries and fried chicken; and the large amounts of fats hidden in foods such as cheese, bacon, baked goods, candy, and ice cream. More on the difference between good and bad fats on page 223, and if you think that you can't take veggies without tons of dressing, turn to page 235 for some tasty salad topping substitutions!

This large pat of butter is about five teaspoons and represents all the added fat you should have each day! The rest should come from your food.

189

Fiber

Fiber is also very important. Although it doesn't provide energy, it does provide a vital service. Fiber is like a Roomba for your rear, scrubbing your insides clean of what's left over after your body has extracted all the nutrients from the food you eat. In other words, it helps you make a healthy poop. Teen girls need about 25-30 grams of fiber each day. For more information on how to get that much, go to page 193.

Foods With No Group

Sweets, sodas, candy, alcohol, fat-based food toppings such as gravy and mayonnaise, and highly processed foods such as hot dogs, are "empty calorie" culprits that aren't classified under any food group. Those foods are loaded with calories, but they lack the growth-promoting, life-sustaining nutrients that our bodies crave. These foods won't help your body grow or thrive, but they will help you gain a lot of excess fat if you eat them often. They're often called "junk" and "fake" foods because empty-calorie foods provide energy, but they lack the nutrients you get from veggies, fruits, and whole grains.

This way of grouping foods doesn't mean that sugar and fat are always bad. You just need to know the difference between healthy and not-so-healthy sources. Sugars and fats from natural foods, such as fruits and vegetables, are great. Sugars and fats from fast food milkshakes and fried potatoes are not so great. Why? For one thing, they are different *kinds* of sugars and fats. (More about the differences on pages 220 and 223.)

Rule of thumb: The more natural the food, the more nutrient-dense it will be. (Nutrient-dense foods have a high level of nutrients per calorie.) So, for example, you get more nutrition from 100 calories of grapes than you get from 100 calories of grape-flavored candy.

Water

Although vitamins and minerals are very important, water is the human body's most essential nutrient. It provides no energy because it contains no calories, but it's more crucial to survival than food is! If you ever find yourself stranded on a desert island, you can survive for three weeks or more without food, but you'll last less than a week without water. While water is found in most foods, you still need to drink at least eight glasses a day to keep your body's cells, muscles, and other tissues hydrated. If you're trying to slim down or tone up, you'll find that drinking plenty of water helps burn fat, prevent bloating, and banish headaches! Hydration affects almost everything in your body, from your skin's softness and your blood's thickness to your ability to poop.

The color of your urine can tell you a lot about your drinking habits. The lighter it is, the more hydrated you are. The darker it is, the more water you need to drink. If you know you're getting your eight glasses a day but your pee is still dark, some vitamin supplements, such as Vitamin C, may be tinting your tinkle. But if your urine is dark because your taste buds can't get used to boring old water, turn to page 201 to see how to fit in your daily fluid fix.

Eating Based on Beliefs

Feeding your body better food is hard enough, but when you already have strict limitations on the food you're allowed to eat, scarfing down the same stuff over and over again can become pretty boring. About 3 percent of American teens are vegetarian, and 1 percent are vegan. Vegans don't eat or use animal products of any kind. Vegetarians don't eat animals, but most do consume some animal products, including honey, eggs, butter, and dairy products. Many vegetarian or vegan people also won't wear leather or fur or use beeswax. Teens who are vegan or vegetarian have to pay careful attention to their food to make sure they get enough protein, iron, calcium, zinc, vitamin D, vitamin B12, and other essentials. If you're cutting calories on a vegetarian or vegan food plan, make sure to include high-quality vegetable protein in your meals; good sources are soy, grains, nuts, seeds, and legumes (beans and lentils). Also make sure to take a multivitamin/mineral supplement that's vegetarian friendly (see page 192 for more on vitamins). The same thing goes for healthy eating when you're keeping kosher, halal, or other eating lifestyles based on your beliefs—get in all the food groups your body needs!

Multivitamins and Other Supplements

Vitamins and minerals ward off sickness and keep individual body parts healthy. Although all parts of the body need vitamins and minerals to function, some body parts have especially high needs for particular ones—for example, calcium for bones and teeth, iron for blood, and vitamin C for healing wounds. The body cannot function properly without vitamins and minerals, and an extreme deficiency can be life threatening.

Your body needs dozens of vitamins and minerals. Also, it's near impossible to keep track of calories, food group servings, AND vitamins and minerals, so multivitamin/mineral supplements take the worry out of planning and record keeping!

As important as vitamins and minerals are, don't think that you can take a magic pill, not eat, and lose lots of weight. Multivitamins/minerals can't replace food because they contain no energy! Also, the body improves its processing of minerals and vitamins when they're consumed with other nutrients found in food (such as the "good fats" in nuts and seeds), so you and your bod are better off if you get most of your minerals and vitamins from food. The supplement? It's just a little extra insurance.

The best multivitamin and mineral supplements:

✿ **Meet your daily needs.** Look for one that provides 100 percent of your daily value of the major vitamins and minerals, instead of 20 percent of one and 200 percent of another. While your body usually flushes out the extra with your pee, in some cases the amounts can be too much, especially for the fat-soluble substances (such as vitamin A) that your body stores. If you can't find a multivitamin/mineral supplement that is right for you, talk to your doctor or school nurse. Visit www.nancyredd.com to see a chart of the vitamins your body needs and what each one does!

✿ **Are marked with a "use before" date.** Vitamins and minerals deteriorate over time and they aren't as effective after their expiration date.

✿ **Say "USP" on the label.** USP stands for U.S. Pharmacopeia, the organization that tests supplements for quality. Don't waste your money on a multivitamin/mineral supplement that hasn't been checked!

Two other supplements to consider:

☆ **Those containing good fats such as omega-3 fatty acids** — To keep your skin soft, your hair shiny, and your insides oiled, and maybe give your brain a boost, flaxseed oil and fish oil are superb supplements. They contain large amounts of the all-important omega-3 fatty acids that your body doesn't manufacture, so you must get them from your food. At one school, test results and reading comprehension improved dramatically after the entire student body took fish oil supplements for three months! If you're allergic to seafood, do not try a fish oil supplement until you've talked to your doctor.

☆ **Fiber** — If you're having problems with your poop, you may not be getting enough fiber. You need between 25-30 grams per day, but you may not be getting enough from your food. Certain breakfast cereals can un-bung you (some offer over half your daily needs in just one serving), and chances are, if you start following your food group serving suggestions, you'll easily get enough fiber to get things going. For example, these naturally fibrous options are delicious and you should include them in your healthy meal plan whether you need extra fiber or not: raspberries (8-9 grams per cup), a small baked potato (4 grams), black beans (10 grams per ½ cup), and pears (4-6 grams per medium pear). With fibrous foods like those, who needs fiber supplements? If you still need a supplement, look for products that contain only psyllium husk; reject packaged "fiber cookies," chemically flavored shakes (expensive and yucky), and any preparation that contains a lot of added sugar or chemicals. Don't purchase any product that's labeled as a laxative unless you're following a doctor's orders. You could end up in a lot of discomfort!

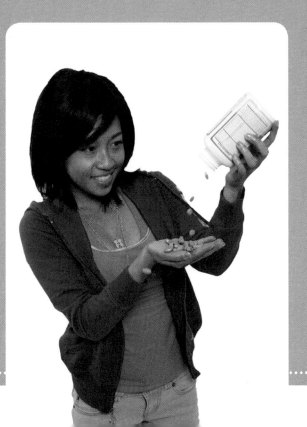

☆ **Steer Clear of ANYTHING ELSE** (unless prescribed by a doctor). Expensive celebrity-endorsed shakes, human growth hormone, protein concoctions, amino acids, creatine, and steroids (duh) aren't good for anyone, but especially not when your body is still developing. Much of the stuff out there isn't tested for safety before it's put on the market. So don't be fooled!

Calcium

You've probably heard a lot about calcium. Young women need LOTS of calcium (1,300+ milligrams per day), and for those of us who are lactose intolerant or who don't own a cow, that amount is difficult to get from food alone.

In 1947, the average American consumed forty gallons of milk and eleven gallons of carbonated soft drinks each year. About fifty years later, milk consumption dropped to twenty-two gallons, while soft drink consumption soared to forty-nine gallons! Our guzzling of soft drinks has more than tripled while our milk drinking has dropped by almost one half. Why is that a problem? Soft drinks are calorie dense and nutrient poor; they provide a lot of sugar (or artificial sweetener) but not much else. Milk, on the other hand, is loaded with nutrients, and it's one of the best sources of the calcium needed for building strong bones and teeth.

After age eighteen, your bones don't get any bigger or longer, but the process of building bone goes on throughout your life. Your bones act as a calcium storehouse and your blood takes calcium from your bones when other parts of your body need it. So calcium is important in the teen years in order to build strong bones; it remains important in adulthood to keep bones strong and supply all parts of the body with the calcium they need.

Perhaps you've heard of the disease osteoporosis, also called "brittle bones." It's rare among young people, but your risk of developing it later in life rises if you don't get enough calcium. To avoid brittle bones, make sure you get your three cups of dairy foods every day, and take a supplement that contains calcium, too. You'll rarely find a multivitamin/mineral pill that meets 100 percent of your calcium needs; it would be too big to swallow! So drink your milk and eat other calcium-rich foods (like broccoli), take a calcium supplement, or invest in a bottle of the popular calcium chews. Also, look for calcium supplements that include magnesium and/or vitamin D. The mixture helps the body absorb calcium better. (In my experience, it also calms you down. Try it. It works for me!)

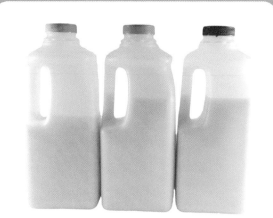

Health Problems and Food

Do some dairy foods blow you up like a balloon? Do peanuts cause your throat to close? Do you have irritable bowel syndrome (IBS)? From lactose intolerance to food allergies to bowel problems, health-related eating issues should be taken seriously. If you have any strange symptoms or discomfort after eating specific substances, whether you've been diagnosed with a food allergy or not, turn to page 242 for gastrointestinal disorders and food allergy resources and see your doctor for help.

BTW: ANEMIA

Are you so busy that you barely have time to breathe? Are you always exhausted or feeling under your game, even when you get plenty of sleep? Do you look pale or feel sickly, even on a good day? Are you a vegetarian? One of the most common nutrient deficiencies among teen girls is iron, which sometimes develops into one form of anemia. Without enough iron, our bodies feel weak, especially when we lose blood, which is how iron travels. So guess what happens to a lot of us who have heavy periods? We become anemic. Vegetarians are at high risk, too, because most iron comes from animal foods (though spinach is a great source). Anemia can often be treated with iron supplements, but what you consume isn't always the culprit, so see your doctor if you suspect that you might be anemic.

Choosing Foods

Don't assume that "low-fat," "low sugar," "fat free," "sugar free," or "reduced calorie" versions of your favorite processed foods are better for you. Often, to improve flavor, companies fill low-fat versions with more sugar and low-sugar snacks with more fat. Read the nutrition labels (see page 212 for how) to decide if you're better off enjoying full-sugar or full-fat versions in smaller portion sizes.

SERVE YOURSELF SMARTLY

Americans typically underestimate the number of calories in the food they eat by 35 percent or more. No wonder we're gaining extra weight! Most of us don't understand the size of a healthy serving. We can't carry a food scale around with us, so being able to eyeball a proper portion size comes in handy. When your portion sizes are under control, fewer extra calories have a chance to sneak through.

Generally speaking, a proper portion of protein, dairy, or grains fits in the palm of your hand (your hand without your fingers or thumb). Portion sizes for fruits and veggies can be a little larger, the size of your entire hand. Those for fats are a whole lot smaller, around the size of a penny (1 teaspoon). But since you can't snatch up steaks and mashed potatoes with your bare hands, it can really help to start thinking about serving sizes in the following ways:

☆ Protein – A serving of meat, poultry, seafood, or tofu (2-3 ounces) is about the size of a deck of cards. If it's the same size as your entire hand including your fingers, then it needs to be thinner or split into two servings.

proper portion
(feels tiny)

oversized portion
(what we're used to)

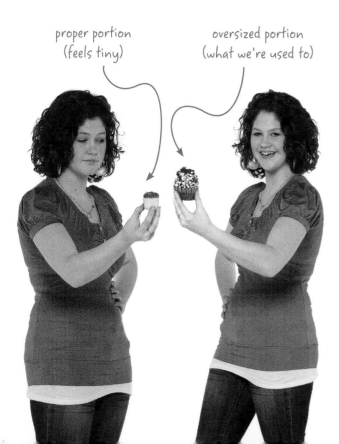

☆ Grains: Cereal, Rice, Pasta – A single serving of cereal, rice, or pasta (1 ounce) is about the same size as an ice cream scoop. A piece of bread that's about the size of your hand, including fingers, is one serving.

☆ Vegetables and Fruits – One handful or the size of your fist is a good estimate of a single serving (1 cup), but unless your plant food has been cooked in oil, sweetened with sugar, or fried, you don't have to be as careful about portion sizes. Many fruits come already "packaged" in natural serving sizes: one orange, one banana, one small apple.

The proper serving size for a baked potato is as the same size as a computer mouse, which—surprise, surprise—was designed to fit into the palm of your hand.

★ Dairy – One individual cup of yogurt or one small individual milk carton is a single serving (1 cup). A cube that's an inch on each side (about the length of the first joint on your finger) is a serving of cheese (1 ounce).

★ Fats – When you use butter, dressings, mayonnaise, or other fats and oils, try to limit each serving to about the size of a penny (1 teaspoon). Using such a small amount of spread may take some getting used to, but your body will love you for it.

Eyeballing portions works well as long as you're choosing foods that haven't been heavily processed and that don't contain a lot of added fat, sugar, or empty calories. So if you're snacking on strawberry fruit gummies instead of fresh strawberries, you'll need to decrease your portion sizes. (See page 208 for more on the benefits of whole foods.) The eyeballing approach also stops working the minute you go back for seconds. Save that second helping for a snack to have later!

Trick Your Eyes

f.y.i.

If you put a handful of food on a huge dinner plate, the portion looks skimpy and you may feel hungry and deprived. Put that same portion on a salad or dessert plate, and you'll feel indulged and satisfied. Try it! It works!

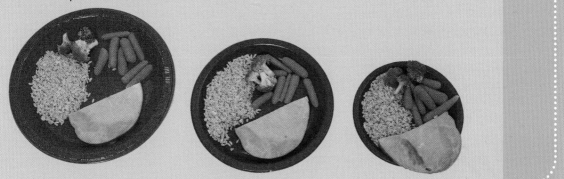

Squeeze In Every Serving

There are several food groups, and it can be tricky to squeeze in the recommended number of servings each day. Luckily, there are a variety of foods in each group, and eating all of the servings you need is doable with a little effort. To help you check off the servings you've already eaten or planned for, try creating a daily food checklist (or visit www.nancyredd.com for a printable version). First, write down all the meals you have in a day, maybe three meals and two snacks. Then, using the number of calories you're eating (turn to page 212 to find out how to read nutrition labels for this information), start plugging in the foods that you eat, checking the box for the covered food group servings as you go. Here is an example of a girl who is eating 1,800 calories per day:

DAILY SERVING CHECKLIST

Protein – 2–3 servings/5 ½–6 ounces ☐oz. ☐oz. ☐oz. ☐oz. ☐oz. ☐oz.

Grains – 6 servings/ounces ☐oz. ☐oz. ☐oz. ☐oz. ☐oz. ☐oz.

Dairy – 3 servings/cups ☐cup ☐cup ☐cup

Veggies – 2–3 servings/cups ☐cup ☐cup ☐cup

Fruit – 2 servings/cups ☐cup ☐cup

Added Fats – no more than 5 teaspoons ☐tsp. ☐tsp. ☐tsp. ☐tsp. ☐tsp.

✰ **BREAKFAST:** 1 7" banana (100 calories of fruit), ½ cup of oatmeal (150 calories of grains) with 1 tablespoon of sugar (30 calories), topped with 17 almonds (1 oz., 120 calories of protein), 1 cup of 2 percent milk (130 calories of dairy) **Total: 530 calories, 1 fruit, 1 grains, 1 protein, 1 dairy**

✰ **SNACK:** 5 whole-wheat crackers (50 calories of grains), 1 ounce of cheese (100 calories of dairy) **Total: 150 calories, 1 grains, 1 dairy**

✰ **LUNCH:** 2 pieces of wheat bread (120 calories of grains), 3 turkey sandwich slices (2.5 oz., 75 calories of protein), 1 teaspoon of mayonnaise (33 calories of added fats), 1 tablespoon of mustard (14 calories), 1 small apple (65 calories of fruit), 1 cup of 2 percent milk (130 calories of dairy) **Total: 450 calories, 2 grains, 2.5 protein, 1 added fat, 1 fruit, 1 dairy**

☆ **SNACK:** 12 baby carrots (50 calories of veggies), 1 tablespoon of natural peanut butter (.5 oz., 100 calories of protein) **Total: 150 calories, 1 veggie, .5 protein**

☆ **DINNER:** 3 oz. of skinless, baked chicken (100 calories of protein), ½ cup cooked brown rice (120 calories of grains), 1 cup of steamed spinach (10 calories of veggies), 1 sweet potato (100 calories of veggies), 1 piece of wheat bread (60 calories of grains), 1 cup of 2 percent milk (130 calories of dairy) **Total: 520 calories, 3 protein, 2 grains, 2 veggie, 1 dairy**

See? When you plan properly, eating all your daily servings within 1,800 calories a day isn't a problem!

BTW: PORTION SIZES HAVE CHANGED!

Baked potatoes as big as your feet, steaks that barely fit on the plate—restaurant portions are out of control! In 1960, a serving of French fries at a fast food restaurant contained 200 calories; today a supersized portion contains nearly three times that. Sodas were once 12 ounces and about 140 calories; now the smallest drink is 16 ounces, but who stops there? Why not go for the "bargain," 64-ounce supergulp at 750 calories—all of them from sugar? It's not hard to eat an entire day's calorie allowance in a single meal. Whereas the average combo used to be an acceptable 590 calories, today it's not uncommon to order feasts of well over 1,500 calories! So think twice before you order. Check the menu for options noted as "healthy" or "light," and don't be ashamed to look to the kiddy menu for portion sizes that make sense for a healthy teen. Regardless of what you order, just because it's on your tray, you don't have to put it into your mouth. Remember the handful rule and split your large servings with a friend or package extra food to take home for two meals for the price of one!

then!

now!

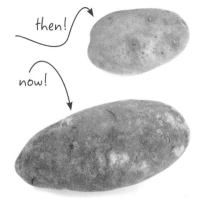

Savvy Snacks

Ninety-eight percent of teens today snack between meals (up from 74 percent in 1977), which should be a good thing for your metabolism and your brain. However, in practice, the calories that most teens are getting from snacks aren't providing much in the way of good nutrition. The most popular snacks are salty, fatty, and sugary junk, including candy, crackers, pretzels, dessert foods, and sweet drinks. If you're trying to feed your body better, here are some simple switches for smarter snacking.

Crunchy
Choose homemade microwave potato chips over potato chips from a bag. Slice a potato or sweet potato paper thin (you may need an adult to help you). Coat a large microwaveable plate with cooking spray and arrange slices in a single layer. Spray slices with cooking spray and cook in the microwave for 3 to 8 minutes until browned slightly. Be careful not to let them burn! Sprinkle with salt, pepper, vinegar, hot sauce, lime juice, or whatever seasonings you like! Your first batch might not be perfect, but once you get the timing right you'll never crave a regular chip again!

Sweet
For a special sweet treat, try freezing grapes. They're better than popsicles!

Salty
Try two or three dill pickles, or a handful of dry roasted pumpkin or sunflower seeds with the shell on.

Tangy
A handful of cherry tomatoes makes a crisp and tangy snack. At only three calories each, you can have quite a few if you're hungry!

Creamy
Try mashing a banana with a little milk and honey. The creaminess factor is out of control! Or if you have an almost overripe banana on hand, peel it and stick it on a plate in the freezer for another awesome treat.

Drink More Water

The smartest swap you can make is choosing water over sodas, fruit drinks, and large amounts of fruit juice. However, some types of water taste better than others, and there are plenty of calorie-free flavor-fixes that will help you down the eight glasses a day you need to stay healthy and hydrated.

✰ **A home water-filter pitcher ($5 per month)** – These contraptions have saved my life. I never knew water could taste so good. Not all of them deliver the same results, though, so if you don't like the first one you try, experiment with a different brand.

✰ **Bottled water ($10-12 per month)** – For under a dollar, your local grocery store probably sells spring water in gallon-sized containers. Some stores have systems that let you purchase a bottle and return it for a refill each time you shop there.

✰ **Carbonated water ($15-20 per month)** – Sparkling water (naturally bubbly) and carbonated water (artificially bubbly) have the same health benefits as flat water but with the party-in-your-mouth feel of soda, and some people think the bubbles improve the flavor. Take care, though. Too much carbonation might make you feel bloated and gassy.

✰ **Low-cost flavor treats** – Try sprucing up your water with a squeeze of lemon juice, a crushed strawberry, or a slice of cucumber. Yum!

Drinks Count!

f.y.i.

Chewing is not a requirement for calories to count! Drinks are food in liquid form, but we tend to overlook them. We often forget to count the calories in our creamy cappuccinos, and we don't notice that liquid calories are much less filling than a solid food of the same calorie count. Avoid sugary sodas and those fancy lattes—some of them contain almost as many calories as you need for an entire day—and replace them with water. You'll notice a difference in everything, from how well you sleep and how blemish-free your skin becomes to how your cellulite lessens on your thighs! Increasing your intake of water to at least eight glasses a day—more if you're still thirsty—is one of the best steps you can take toward improving your health.

WHAT 100-CALORIE PORTIONS LOOK LIKE

With all this talk about calorie counts, servings, handfuls, scoops, and decks of cards, why do you need to know what 100-calories portions look like? For a variety of reasons. First, comparing 100 calories of vegetables to 100 calories of candy (for example, the tomatoes and the caramel cups pictured on page 170) will help you understand the difference between nutrient-dense foods (the tomatoes) and calorie-dense foods (the caramel cups). Second, when you become aware of the amounts of food that contribute 100 calories to your daily total, you'll do better at estimating and controlling your portion sizes. Knowing what 100-calorie quantities look like will help you to make the most of your daily calories. Which looks more satisfying, 100 calories of caramel cups or 100 calories of tomatoes?

Lettuce = 1 whole head (10 servings)

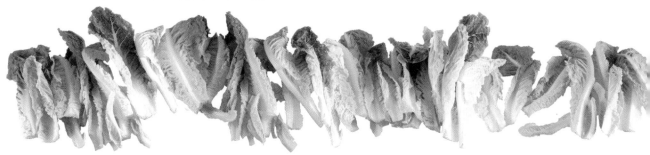

Dill Pickles = 21 3" pickles (7 servings)

Orange Juice = 8 ounces
100% juice (1 serving)

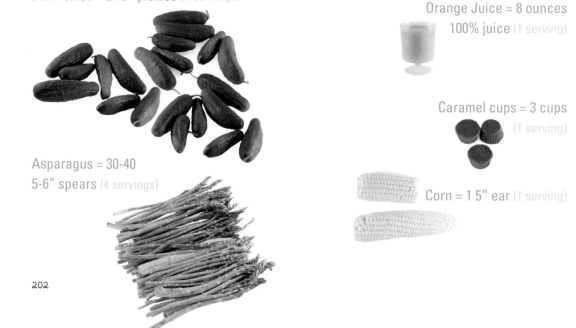

Caramel cups = 3 cups
(1 serving)

Asparagus = 30-40
5-6" spears (4 servings)

Corn = 1 5" ear (1 serving)

202

Cucumbers = 5 6" cucumbers (7 servings)

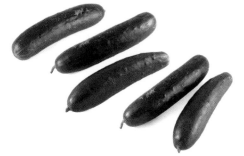

Broccoli = 25 Flowerettes (4 servings)

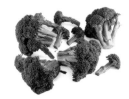

Licorice Candy – 2.5 pieces (1 serving)

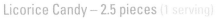

Cauliflower = 4 cups (4 servings)

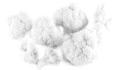

Carrots = 3 9" carrots (3 servings)

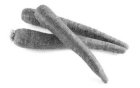

Tomatoes = 6 2.5" tomatoes (3 servings)

Sweet Potato = 1 5" sweet potato (1 serving)

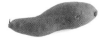

Potato = 1 1.5"-diameter potato (1 serving)

Zucchini = 2.5 6" zucchinis (2.5 servings)

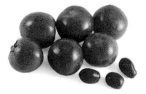

Strawberries = 15 2"-diameter
strawberries (2 servings)

Raisins = about 65 raisins (2 servings)

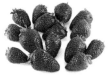
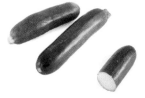

Potato Chips = 10-11 chips (1 serving)

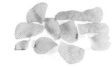
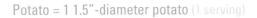

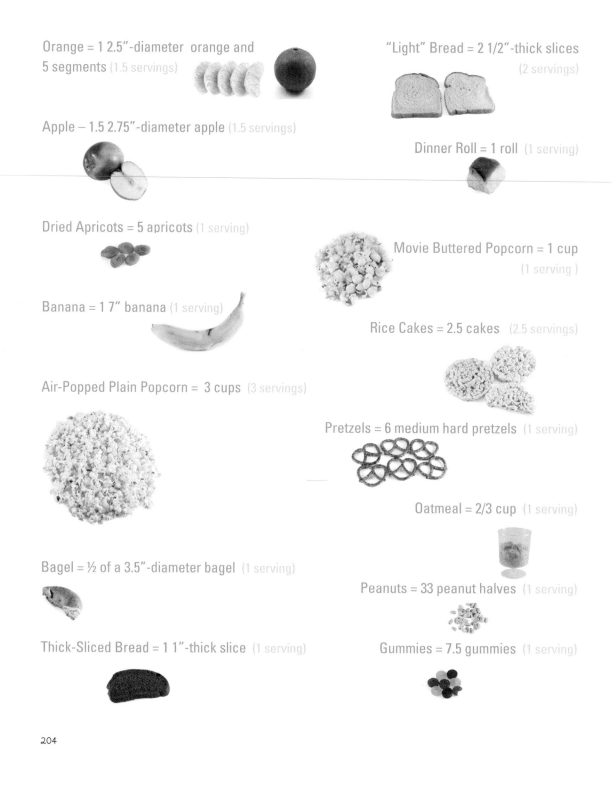

Orange = 1 2.5"-diameter orange and 5 segments (1.5 servings)

"Light" Bread = 2 1/2"-thick slices (2 servings)

Apple – 1.5 2.75"-diameter apple (1.5 servings)

Dinner Roll = 1 roll (1 serving)

Dried Apricots = 5 apricots (1 serving)

Movie Buttered Popcorn = 1 cup (1 serving)

Banana = 1 7" banana (1 serving)

Rice Cakes = 2.5 cakes (2.5 servings)

Air-Popped Plain Popcorn = 3 cups (3 servings)

Pretzels = 6 medium hard pretzels (1 serving)

Oatmeal = 2/3 cup (1 serving)

Bagel = ½ of a 3.5"-diameter bagel (1 serving)

Peanuts = 33 peanut halves (1 serving)

Thick-Sliced Bread = 1 1"-thick slice (1 serving)

Gummies = 7.5 gummies (1 serving)

Animal Crackers = 11 crackers (1 serving)

Skim Milk =
        10 ounces (1.2 servings)

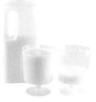

1% Milk = 8 ounces
(1 serving)

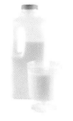

Whole Milk = 5.5 ounces
            (3/5 of a serving)

Cream = 2 tablespoons
(1 serving)

Beans = a little less than ½ cup (1 serving)

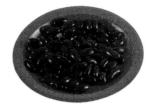

Pasta = 23-25 1.5" pieces (1 serving)

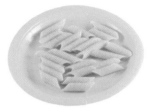

Steamed Shrimp= 7 pieces (1 serving)

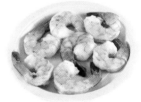

Fried Shrimp = 3 pieces
(1 serving)

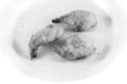

**Depending on the size, shape, weight, and manufacturer of your food,
your calorie counts may vary, so use this information as a guide and not as a set given!**

You FEED Your Body When You...
CARE ABOUT WHAT YOU CONSUME

OK, let's keep it real. When you go from being clueless about nutrition to feeding your body nothing but healthy food 95 percent of the time, the journey isn't a short skip. It's a giant leap! As I sit here typing away, craving yet another chocolate chip cookie that I can't fit into today's calorie count (I've already had two today and it's only two o'clock in the afternoon), I am NOT going to pretend that eating healthily is an easy change or even a quick one.

What you can do immediately, however, is to start caring about the quality of what you consume. Begin by paying attention to whether your food choices are helping you reach your goals, whether you want to slim down or simply promote good health. When you care, it's easier to say no to that third cookie and reach instead for a handful of cherry tomatoes, as I'm doing as I write. Why? Because you and I know that we're not punishing ourselves; we are improving ourselves and taking good care of our bodies!

fast fact

Thirty years ago, a visit to a fast food restaurant was a rare treat. Today, one out of every four Americans eats fast food every day. On any given day, 30 percent of American teens eat fast food at least once! Although nearly every fast food restaurant offers healthy options on the menu, most customers choose chicken nuggets, hamburgers, French fries, milk shakes, fried apple pies, and other goodies-to-go. Be different!

Caring about what you consume means that you take time to think about what you're putting in your body, not only by eating the right number of servings from all the food groups, but also by paying attention to what's in the food you eat. One hundred years ago, no one worried about how their foods had been processed or modified; nearly all of the foods available were "whole foods," meaning they came directly from the ground or an animal. But today, many foods have been cooked, canned, frozen, bottled, dehydrated, pressed, pureed, or preserved—and some unpronounceable ingredients have often been added to them. It pays to know what to look for and avoid!

Whole, "unprocessed" foods have had nothing added or removed from them, keeping them healthy and nutritious. You'll find whole foods in the produce, meat, dairy, and seafood departments at your grocery store and on the cereal and rice/beans aisles, too (if you select the lightly processed kinds). Whole foods are typically better for you because the more a food is processed, the less nutritious it becomes. Microwave-ready meals, boxed and packaged "dinners," and fast-cooking convenience foods may save time, but at what price? Some of them serve up longer expiration dates and more addictive tastes (added fat, sugar, and salt) at the expense of good nutrition.

If we ate only whole foods, we wouldn't need to worry about nutrition labels or learn the lingo of preservatives, additives, and processes, nor would our society have nearly the number of health and obesity problems that we do. But processed foods are now so cheap and readily available—and we've grown so accustomed to the taste and the convenience in our hurry-up lifestyles—that today close to 90 percent of the typical American family's food budget is spent on processed foods. So if you're eating frozen dinners, packaged lunch meats, instant pasta dishes, and lots of other things that come from boxes and cans, chances are you're not getting enough of the nutrients that you need, even if you "look healthy" and are ticking off all of the recommended servings and food groups!

Processed foods aren't going away anytime soon, so it's up to us to care enough to check out ingredients and make the best choices possible about what we consume. The best way to start caring is by learning to read and understand nutrition labels. Turn to page 212 to find out how.

Processed vs. Whole Foods

I've advised you to eat whole foods, and half of your grains are supposed to be whole grains, but what does "whole" mean?

Various methods of refining or processing are used to preserve foods or make them safer. Pasteurization is an example of a simple refining process that makes milk safe to drink. But today many foods are more than lightly processed. They are prepared ahead of time to cook faster, look better, or last longer on the shelf. Why is flour bleached white? No reason, except that it stores longer and looks "pretty."

When it comes to the nutrient value of foods we eat, it often IS what's on the outside that counts. When skins and shells are removed, fiber and nutrients are lost. For example, removing the husks and polishing rice makes it attractive and longer lasting, but the process removes a lot of the nutrition that was in the original brown rice. Still other refining and processing happens during cooking, as when foods are boiled and then canned, losing many nutrients in the process. While some snack foods, refined foods, and sodas are fortified with vitamins (a fancy way of saying that vitamins are added in), your body prefers getting its nutrients through healthy, whole foods.

Here are a few common refined and/or processed foods and the best substitutions for them that you can make.

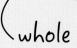

whole

processed

PROCESSED/REFINED	WHOLE
White rice (polished to remove the outer layer, along with 60-100 percent of the vitamins and fiber)	Brown rice
White flour (bleached until 80 percent of the vitamins and minerals and 75 percent of the fiber are gone)	Whole-wheat flour and the things made from it, such as breads and pastas
Table sugar (stripped of almost all vitamins, minerals, and fiber in the process of turning cane juice into white sugar); the leader in the "empty calories" division (see page 190)	Honey, molasses, 100% percent pure maple syrup (in small amounts)
Quick-cook oats (processed so that many nutrients are lost through the steaming and toasting process)	Old-fashioned or steel-cut oats
Chicken nuggets (ground chicken scraps mixed with water, fats, chemicals, and spices, breaded, and fried into tiny balls that are so common many kids think are healthy and natural, not knowing that no part of a real chicken resembles a nugget)	Baked, whole, skinless chicken breasts, legs, and thighs, with or without a cornflake or breadcrumb coating
Anything canned (heated to high temperatures to sterilize and preserve. The heat can break down some of the nutrients in the food. Canned foods often contain preservatives, fats, and sugars that are added for "flavor.") Canned soups usually suffer from sodium overload.	Fresh or frozen foods with no sugars or fats added. If you must buy canned soups, look for ones that are low sodium.
Anything sweetened (like applesauce) or with "extra flavor"	Unsweetened products and those without added flavorings

Diabetes

Have you heard that there are two types of diabetes, but you don't know the difference? Type 1 is inherited, and it cannot be prevented. It usually begins in childhood or the early teen years; it is treated with insulin because the body does not produce enough. Only about 10 percent of people with diabetes have type 1.

The other 90 percent have type 2 diabetes. With Type 2, the body still makes insulin, but cells become resistant to its effects. That means that muscles don't take up the sugar they need for energy, so the level of glucose in the blood rises, affecting and damaging all the body's organs. Although symptoms include blurred vision, fatigue, frequent thirst, and frequent peeing, one third of people with type 2 diabetes have no idea they have the disease! Diabetes can

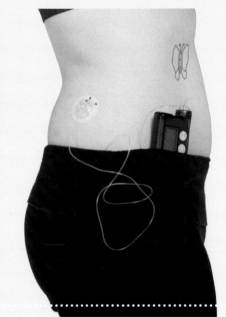

shorten your life, especially if left untreated, so it's important to ask your doctor for a blood glucose test to check for the disease (see page 56).

Many factors increase the risk of developing type 2 diabetes, among them—you guessed it—too little exercise and too much body weight. That's why more young people are now getting type 2, which used to be a disease of older people. Numbers are growing so rapidly each year that experts now predict that 40 percent of females will develop type 2 diabetes sometime in their lives!

Those predictions are based on current trends, but we can change those numbers if we get off the couch and start eating right and exercising!

belly laughs

My doctor told me about a call she received:

"I'm diabetic and I might have had too much sugar today. How can I tell?" the terrified teen asked.

"Well, first off, are you light-headed?" my doctor quizzed.

"No," the teen snapped. "I'm a brunette."

Success Story: Kim

"Being overweight was something I didn't think would ever change for me. My mom was a big woman, and I was ten pounds eight ounces at birth, so I was big from the beginning. Throughout my younger years, I was heavy, and I was always made fun of. When I was a kid, my family and friends would constantly comment on my weight, which made me feel self-conscious, embarrassed, and excluded.

"Finally, when I was thirteen, my mom decided to stop being unhealthy and she wanted me to join her. At first, I wasn't sure, but I kinda had no choice. She did all the cooking, so whatever healthy meals she started making for herself she made for me, and there was nothing else to eat! When I saw the results, I became so enthusiastic that I started turning down junk food at school and at friends' houses, too. Then, my mom started doing aerobics tapes at home, so I copied her and did them, too. It started to become fun and over the next year, we not only shaped up but also spent more time together, bonding and talking more even when we weren't exercising.

"She confessed that she'd been cooking unhealthy food and not exercising before because she had been at a low point in her life. But that had changed and she was feeling better and she wanted me to feel good about my body, too. I admire her so much for being so honest and hardworking. I began to feel more confident about more than just my appearance because I could finally run up a flight of stairs, I wasn't picked last to be on teams in gym class, and I got more compliments. In one school year I went from being tormented and teased to being voted best looking, most likely to succeed, and best smile.

"I'm happy with where I am and I do the best I can to maintain my health. To stay in shape I run track and participate in several other activities at my high school. I take the time to make and eat delicious, healthy snacks and meals. It's not hard at all. Apples dipped in honey are tastier than candy, hummus is much better than mayo on bread, and since I'm a choc-o-holic, instead of a chocolate bar with no health benefits I treat myself to a tablespoon of Nutella on whole-grain bread almost every morning. I also indulge in fresh fruit and lowfat chocolate milk. It's the best breakfast ever. It keeps me going and more than satisfies my sweet tooth.

"My number one rule is to stay away from things that contain too much salt. Excess sodium bloats your belly and it's bad for your health! My mom wishes she had cut back on salt before she developed high blood pressure, which, along with diabetes, runs in my family. I used to eat a lot of salty stuff, but now, I can taste the tiniest bit of salt in everything, and so many of the salty foods that I loved when I was unhealthy taste gross to me now!"

LEARN TO READ LABELS

Most foods either come in a package with a nutrition label on it, or nutrition facts are easily found online—even for fast foods. Nutrition labels may seem confusing at first. So much information is squeezed into a such a small space that you may wonder where to begin, but after you decipher a nutrition label once, you'll find that all labels contain the same kinds of information, and you'll learn quickly how to figure out the key nutritional features of any food!

Let's get started with a side-by-side comparison of nutrition labels for two similar, but slightly different, food items so that you can see how the information on the label can affect what you choose to eat.

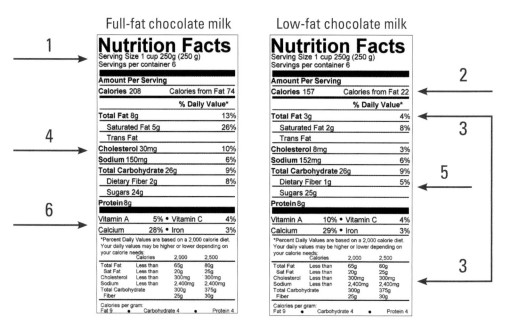

Full-fat chocolate milk

Low-fat chocolate milk

Step 1) Check out the serving size and the number of servings in the package or container. In these examples, the serving size is the same (1 cup) and the number of servings is the same (6). The serving size is important. If you consume two servings instead of one, you take in twice as many calories. For some foods this is easy to understand, but for other foods it can be misleading. When you buy a jar of peanut butter, for example, you know it contains multiple servings, but how many should you have and how much in each one? If you are used to slathering a thick layer of peanut butter on your bread, you may be surprised to find that the serving size is only two tablespoons (at 200 calories). That jar that normally lasts you for only ten sandwiches actually contains fifteen servings! And what about that single muffin that looks like one serving? Read the label and you may find that the manufacturer decided to split that one muffin into two servings and print half the number of calories on the package. That sneaky tactic can mess you up if you're counting calories or watching your fat or sodium levels, so be sure to pay attention not only to the serving size, but also to the number of servings in the package!

Step 2) Look at the number of calories in a serving and the number of calories from fat.
The number of calories tells you how much energy is in one serving of the food. If you are trying to maintain good health or slim down, comparing calorie counts is a good place to start. In these examples, a serving of the low-fat chocolate milk contains fewer calories (157) than the full-fat version (208), which is generally a good thing. (Be careful, however, of foods that substitute artificial sweeteners and fat substitutes as a way of lowering calories. To look for them, check the ingredients list, also on the label. While such additives probably aren't harmful in small amounts, consuming large amounts may not be wise.)

On the same line as "calories," notice the "calories from fat" entry. That number answers the question, "Of all the calories in one serving of this food, how many of them come from fat?" Experts suggest that fat should contribute 30 percent of the calories in a healthy meal plan for teens. On these labels, the whole chocolate milk gets 36 percent (74/208) of its calories from fat. The low-fat milk gets 14 percent (22/157).

Step 3) Study the percent daily values.
The percent daily values on the nutrition label tell you how much of your daily requirement for a nutrient is met by a single serving of the food. If you're eating 2,000 calories every day, you're in luck, because that's the basis for comparison that's used in calculating the percentages (keep reading if you are eating more or less). The percent daily values on the label can help you estimate whether a food will give you enough muscle-building protein and healthy fiber, while keeping excess fat, sugar, or salt (sodium) to a minimum.

Step 4) Look for things you need to limit, like cholesterol, sodium, and "bad" (trans) fats.

Calories come from three basic sources: carbohydrates, fats, and proteins. These substances are different chemically and they perform different functions in the body, but they all contain calories, and any excess over what's burned is stored as fat. The nutrient section of the table shows you the amounts of these basic nutrients in the food, along with additional information on cholesterol and the various kinds of fats, as well as sodium (salt). Here is where you can see a big difference between these two types of milk. The low-fat kind has less saturated fat and cholesterol, while providing the same amount of protein and carbohydrates. The amount of sodium and sugar is a little greater in the low-fat kind and the amount of fiber is a little less, but these small changes don't outweigh the health benefits of reduced fat and cholesterol. Notice the entries for the particular kinds of fats: saturated and trans fats. They are the "bad fats" we try to avoid (see page 223 for more). The low-fat version of the milk contains less saturated fat. Luckily, neither of these milks has any trans fat, which is the worst kind of all (turn to page 223 to find out why).

Step 5) Look at the fiber content.

Teen girls need about 25-30 grams of fiber each day to keep things moving nicely, and keeping a tally through nutrition labels makes it easy to see if you're missing the mark or are right on target with your fiber needs. Seeing that neither of these milks contributes a lot of fiber reminds you that you need to eat your fruits, whole grains, and veggies to get enough!

Step 6) See what other nutrients the food provides.

While you don't need to worry about this section if you are balancing your plate and taking a multivitamin/mineral supplement, these numbers can give you a good idea of the nutritional value of a food. Milk, for example, is a great source of calcium and vitamin A. In general, the higher the percentage of daily values of nutrients shown in this section of the label, the healthier the food choice.

Regarding the percent daily values, what if you are eating more or less than 2,000 calories a day, but you want to know your recommended daily values? The percents for cholesterol, sodium, vitamins, and minerals—which do not contribute calories—remain the same no matter what your calorie intake. The other percents, however, are based on total calories consumed. So, the percents of daily values for the energy-giving nutrients are always calculated this way:

- ☆ total fat: up to 30% of calories
- ☆ saturated fat: up to 10% of calories
- ☆ carbohydrate: 60% of calories
- ☆ protein: 10% of calories

So, suppose you are consuming 1,600 calories a day. What should your total fat intake be? Since total fat should provide around 30 percent of your calories for good brain development, about 480 of your daily calories should come from fat. (That's about 53 grams of fat, because each gram of fat contains 9 calories). Fewer than 18 of those grams (160 calories) should be saturated fat. Aim for a trans fat intake that's as close to zero as you can manage.

Here's another example: You need protein for growth and strength. If you're eating 1,800 calories a day, 180 of those calories should come from protein. Protein has 4 calories per gram, so you need about 45 grams of protein. One cup of the lowfat chocolate milk shown in the label would provide 8 grams of protein, or about 18 percent (8/45) of your daily need.

BTW: SALT

Americans are addicted to salt, and we're only partly to blame. Processed foods and restaurant meals account for 80 percent of the salt in our foods, and some powerful groups, such as the Institute of Medicine, are pressuring food companies and the government to reduce the amount of salt that can be added to food. Food companies are resisting, however, because people often say they don't like the taste of low-salt foods. Physicians counter that cutting salt could save 150,000 lives a year, primarily because too much salt contributes to high blood pressure in some people. Such individuals should consume no more than 1,500 milligrams a day. If you're sticking to mostly whole foods, you can probably stay healthy by eating less than 2,300 milligrams of salt daily.

LEARN FOOD LINGO

Now that you have cracked the nutrition label code, the next place you should always look is the ingredients list, which is also on the package or on the food producer's Web site. If you compare brands of the same food, you may find large differences in ingredients, depending on how the food is processed. Take, for example, my favorite peanut butter from a local health food store, a popular brand's "natural" version, and a "regular" version of the same brand:

Health food brand	Popular brand's natural version	Popular brand's regular version
Ingredients: Organic peanuts, salt	Ingredients: Roasted peanuts, sugar, palm oil, salt, molasses	Ingredients: Peanuts, sugar, molasses, fully hydrogenated vegetable oils, mono- and diglycerides, salt

These ingredient lists are great examples of how even a food product as simple as peanut butter can contain many added ingredients you might not expect. Don't assume that "natural" versions are any better until you read the labels. Sometimes they are processed almost exactly the same way and simply sold at a higher price!

Until now, if you even looked at the ingredients list on your favorite foods, you probably glossed over the words you didn't understand, and that may have been most of them. But what

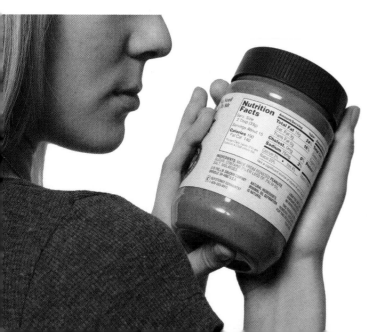

you don't know CAN hurt you! The regular peanut butter, for example, contains hydrogenated vegetable oils, which are one of the worst kind of bad fats.

Ingredients appear in order of weight, meaning the heaviest, most prominent ingredient appears first and the lightest and least ingredient appears last in the lineup. Notice that the second ingredient in both the "natural" and the "regular" peanut butters is sugar. It's added to make the peanut butter taste good, but what if you're trying to limit sugars? You may be getting more sugar than you want. When you start caring about feeding your body with the best food you can—whether you're shopping the snack aisle, the produce section, or the ice cream freezer—you look for foods that contain the healthiest ingredients. That's a choice that anyone can make!

As for those unpronounceable ingredients, they are *food additives*. The higher up the list they appear, the greater their relative amount in the food. Food manufacturers are quick to point out that the substances they add to food are generally considered safe. Additives preserve or improve taste and appearance. Some additives keep food from spoiling before it

fast fact

Do you want to look up nutritional information for your favorite foods? Visit www.nancyredd.com for a list of online nutrition label resources.

hits the stores or your stomach. But do those additives promote good health? Many additives contain chemicals that have been linked to cancer, but they're still in some of our favorite foods!

So it's smart to shop for foods labeled:

✫ NO ADDITIVES   ✫ NO ADDED SALT

✫ NO PRESERVATIVES   ✫ NO ARTIFICIAL FLAVORS

✫ NO ADDED SUGAR   ✫ NO ARTIFICIAL COLORS

If such statements are nowhere to be seen, check the ingredient list for these additives:

✫ Red dye #3 and (perhaps) some other food dyes. Some food dyes have been linked to increases in particular kinds of cancer, but the dyes are still found in candies, gelatins, various drinks, and even those bright red maraschino cherries that look so pretty in a drink. While tiny amounts may not cause a serious problem, if you have a choice between uncolored or colored foods, go for the uncolored.

✫ Sodium nitrate and sodium nitrite. Don't confuse these compounds with ordinary table salt (sodium chloride). They are found naturally in many foods, but they are also added as preservatives to a lot of cured meats, including hot dogs, sausages, ham, and bacon. Some studies have linked these substances to an increased risk of cancer. The reason is that cancer-causing substances called nitrosamines can form when the food is heated or digested.

✦ Sulfites. These compounds are often used to prevent discoloration in dried food such as raisins and apricots, and they are also added to wine. Some people are sensitive to sulfites, which can cause headaches, hives, sneezing—even difficulty breathing. The labels of some brands of dried fruit say "sulfite-free" for that reason.

✦ Butylated hydroxyanisole (BHA) & butylated hydrozyttoluene (BHT). These additives keep fats and oils from spoiling, but debate over their (possibly serious) health effects rages. At this point, it's hard to say if they are safe. Watch to see what new research reveals in the years to come.

✦ Monosodium glutamate (MSG). Found in restaurant fare and many packaged items—including potato chips, frozen foods, and salad dressings—MSG isn't only in Asian foods. It's used widely as a flavor enhancer. Although nothing has been proven, some people say they are sensitive to MSG claiming it causes numbness, tingling, flushing, headaches, and drowsiness. Although MSG is generally recognized as safe, you may want to look for it in the ingredients list if you think you are sensitive to it.

✦ Partially hydrogenated or hydrogenated fats and oils. These are code words for trans fats, which are the worst type of fat. They are found in fried foods, vegetable shortenings, hard margarine, and processed cookies, crackers, cakes, pies, and chips. Consuming hydrogenated fats greatly increases the risk of heart disease, and some experts and individuals are working hard to get them removed from our food supply. You can remove them from yours by looking at labels!

☆ High-fructose corn syrup (HFCS). HFCS is a cheap way to preserve and sweeten foods (and improve the taste of foods that aren't sweet). Evidence is mounting that HFCS is bad for the body. For example, one study showed that it causes greater weight gain, compared to ordinary sugar, even when calorie intake is the same. Although the food industry disputes such research, nutritionists warn that regularly consuming HFCS can lead to obesity, which increases the risk of type 2 diabetes, high blood pressure, and heart disease. Turn to page 220 for more on other added sugars that aren't great for you either.

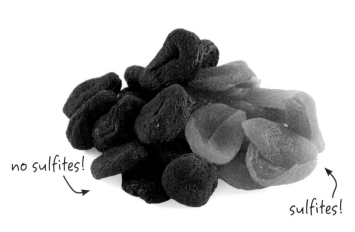

no sulfites!

sulfites!

(They taste the same!)

BTW:

NATURAL DOESN'T MEAN ORGANIC

Don't confuse **natural** with **organic.** Many "natural" foods contain added sugars, fats, flavor enhancers, and more that come from plant or animal sources. The term **organic,** however, means something more. To earn that label, a food must have been produced without using pesticides, hormones, irradiation, genetic engineering, antibiotics, or sewer-sludge or synthetic fertilizers. That's a pretty tough thing to do, so those who are able to produce organic foods can charge higher prices.

SUGAR AND SWEETENERS

ADDED SUGAR SURPRISES

The average teen girl consumes twenty-six teaspoons of sugar a day; the recommended maximum is six! (The natural sugars in fruits, vegetables, and dairy products don't count.) You're probably not throwing your head back and guzzling table sugar, but that doesn't mean you're not overdoing it. Sugar is added to nearly every processed food we consume, even foods that don't taste sweet. When you start looking at ingredients lists, don't be surprised if you see added sugar where you least expect it: in soups, salad dressings, vegetables, crackers, bread, and a lot more. Americans have been hooked on sugar for so long that food manufacturers are afraid we won't like their foods without added sugar, but I say they're not giving us the chance! Many of us feel better when we eliminate added sugar from our food and stick to fruits and dairy products for our sugar highs.

What happens to our bodies when we eat all that excess sugar? Blood sugar levels skyrocket and then plummet, causing mood swings, headaches, exhaustion, stress, irritability, and trouble concentrating—not to mention an increased risk of type 2 diabetes. Oh, and if you don't brush your teeth immediately after eating, you'll be more likely to develop cavities and gum disease, too.

You can take a few simple steps to reduce the amount of added sugar you eat:

☆ Read the ingredients list on food labels. If sugar (or one of its aliases, see page 221) is one of the first three or four ingredients, consider skipping the food or trying a sugarless

fast fact

Fruit-flavored drinks (orange soda, cherry, punch, lemonade, etc.) have hardly any nutritional value and are full of sugar. The same goes for most juices, actually. Unless the juice says "100% juice" on the label (not "100% natural," see page 219 for why), leave it on the shelf.

fast fact

If you find yourself having to sweeten your food with more than a few packets or spoonfuls of sweetener, see your doctor. Sometimes a craving for sweets is a sign of an illness of a lack of essential nutrients.

fast fact

Brown sugar is usually just white sugar with molasses mixed in, so it's no healthier than white sugar.

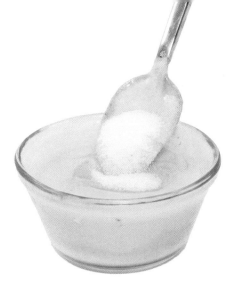

alternative. Love chewing gum? The sugar-free varieties that contain xylitol actually fight tooth decay.

☆ Limit sugary sodas or switch to diet or sugar-free sodas. Better yet, drink water and low-fat milk.

☆ Choose canned fruit packed in water and not syrup. Better yet, eat fresh fruit or frozen fruit without added sugar.

☆ Look for fruit juice that says "100 percent juice." Those that say "100 percent natural" are trying to trick you because, yes, sugar is indeed a natural food. Whatever juice you choose, don't drink a lot of it. Eat the whole fruit instead.

☆ Buy unsweetened ketchup, peanut butter, cereals, yogurt, and jams. You might not like the taste at first but once your taste buds get used to less sugar, you'll never go back to the oversweetened versions. If you want to add a little sweetness, sprinkle on your own sugar or artificial sweetener. Amounts are easier to control when you take charge!

BTW:
ADDED SUGAR ALIASES

Sugar goes by many names. Honey and molasses you probably already know about, but watch for the word **sugar** after "table, white, brown, confectioner's, raw, powdered, and beet." Learn to recognize these ingredients as sugar, too, if you see them on a food label:
- syrup (maple, rice, malt, corn, etc.)
- cane anything (juice, sweetener, syrup, etc.)
- corn anything (juice, sweetener, syrup, etc.)
- fructose, dextrose, glucose, lactose, maltose, sucrose (While these sugars are natural, they needn't be added to foods— but they are.)

Artificial Sweeteners

Although they aren't on the DO NOT EVER EAT lists, the reputation of artificial sweeteners isn't completely clean. We've all heard the scary gossip: Do artificial sweeteners cause cancer? Do they kill brain cells? Do they make you fat? The answer is no, but some people do complain about artificial sweeteners causing headaches, bloating, and other body bummers, especially when they are overused. Also, some people don't like the taste of artificial sweeteners, but there are many varieties, so you may want to try some if you have a sweet tooth!

Artificial sweeteners, also known as sugar substitutes, are natural or manmade compounds that taste sweet but have fewer calories than sugar. They are probably fine when used in moderation (meaning not too often), and they're a good substitute for sugar if you're trying to cut down on calories. Many artificial sweeteners actually taste sweeter than sugar—gram for gram—so you need less to produce a sweet flavor.

Common ones include:

Name	Brands	Can you cook with it?	Is it natural?
Aspartame	NutraSweet, Equal (also contains other ingredients)	No	No
Saccharin	SugarTwin, Sweet'N Low (also contains natural dextrose)	Yes	No
Sucralose	Splenda	Yes	Kinda—it is made from sugar
Stevia	Stevia	Yes	Yes
Luo Han Guo	Luo, Han Guo, numerous brands	Yes	Yes
Xylitol	Xylitol, numerous brands	Yes	Yes

FATS AND OILS

GOOD FATS, BAD FATS

Fats have gotten a bum rap because of trans and saturated fats, but eating good fat is the only way that our bodies can absorb certain important nutrients. Our bodies need fat. Fat protects organs from damage, maintains the membranes around cells, and stores the body's reserves of some important vitamins. Fat is essential for normal sexual development and reproduction, too. Our bodies store extra calories as fat, giving us a long-term energy source that's available in case we can't get food.

For brain development, teen girls need 30 percent of their daily calories to come from fats, preferably healthy fats including unsaturated (also called monounsaturated and polyunsaturated) vegetable oils and the omega-3 fatty acids found in certain fish and some plant foods (see page 224 for more). These healthy fats keep your body working well. They actually *decrease* your risk of developing heart disease!

However, two other major kinds of fats, saturated and trans fat, are harmful to your health, increasing your risk of heart disease. You may need a little time to get over your fear of fats and learn to tell the good from the bad, but it's important that you try. On the next page is a list so you know what to look for when you're food shopping.

Cholesterol

Our bodies naturally produce cholesterol, a type of fat, but we also consume it in certain foods. There are two types of cholesterol in your body: good and bad. Good cholesterol (also called HDL) latches onto the bad (also called LDL and VLDL) and pushes it out of the body, but when there's more bad than good, the good cholesterol becomes overwhelmed and the bad cholesterol stays put, choosing to make its home in the arteries and increasing the risk of heart disease or a heart attack.

Some people inherit genes that cause their bodies to make too much cholesterol. High levels of bad cholesterol (and other bad fats in the blood) are not just an adult problem; 20 percent of teens test too high for one or more of them. Although no one is immune, cutting down on harmful fats in food, feeding your body from all of the food groups, and getting a lot of exercise will lower your risk of heart disease. Turn to page 56 to find out how to get your cholesterol level tested.

f.y.i.

GREEN LIGHT
GO FOR IT!
Healthy Polyunsaturated and
Monounsaturated Fats
Sources include:
> nuts and seeds
> avocados
> olive oil
> canola oil
> peanut oil

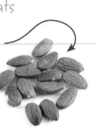

GREEN LIGHT
GO FOR IT!
Healthy Omega-3
Fatty Acids
Sources include:
> salmon, mackerel, tuna, and herring
> flaxseed and flaxseed oil
> walnuts
> canola oil

YELLOW LIGHT
CAUTION: LIMIT AMOUNTS!
Unhealthy Saturated Fat
Sources include:
> red meat (especially if it hasn't been
>   trimmed of most fat)
> poultry that hasn't been skinned
> egg yolks
> butter and shortening
> heavy cream
> ice cream
> full-fat milk

RED LIGHT
STOP: DON'T EAT THESE!
Unhealthy Trans Fats
Sources include:
> store-bought baked goods (cookies,
>   cakes, pies, crackers) that don't say
>   they're 100 percent trans-fat free
> fried foods
> some ice creams
> some restaurant food
> margarine
> some salad dressings

Notice anything contradictory? Healthy food sources such as meat and chicken can contain unhealthy saturated fats. But you can cut your intake of unhealthy fats by taking the skin off poultry, trimming the fat on meats, removing the yolk when eating eggs, using olive oil when cooking instead of butter or shortening, and substituting low-fat milk for full-fat milk or cream.

Frequent Food Mistakes

Even though you now know how to read labels, many of us might assume without looking that these choices are better for us, but they're not!

✩ **Salad covered in dressing instead of a burger and fries.** While still processed and full of preservatives, a regular burger and a small order of fries (like the kind you'd get in a kids' meal) is only about 480 calories and 20 grams of fat. While a grilled chicken salad on its own has less than half the fat and calories (220 calories, 6 grams of fat), the packet of dressing that is included carries with it an additional 190 calories and 18 grams of fat, meaning this meal has more fat and almost the same number of calories! The best thing to do is to learn to love the salad without the dressing (or with smaller quantities of low-fat dressings), or choose healthier toppings (see page 235).

✩ **Assuming "grilled chicken" means "good for you."** Oftentimes, grilled restaurant food is basted with so much oil that it's higher in fat and calories than red meat! Great example: the grilled chicken sandwich at a very popular fast food restaurant has 420 calories and 10 grams of fat, which is way more than the regular hamburger or even the cheeseburger!

Always check the nutrition facts of your favorite "health" foods before blindly picking foods that sound healthier but aren't!

BTW : FEW THINGS IN LIFE ARE (FAT) FREE

The peanut butter on page 216 lists a trans fat alias in the ingredients list (hydrogenated vegetable oils), but the nutrition label shows no trans fat. How? If a serving contains less than 0.5 grams of any nutrient the company legally doesn't have to list it. But serving sizes on labels can be small, so suppose you chow down on four servings, each of which contains 0.4 grams of hidden trans fats. You've accidentally eaten 1.6 grams of the stuff! Pay attention not just to nutrition labels but also to ingredients.

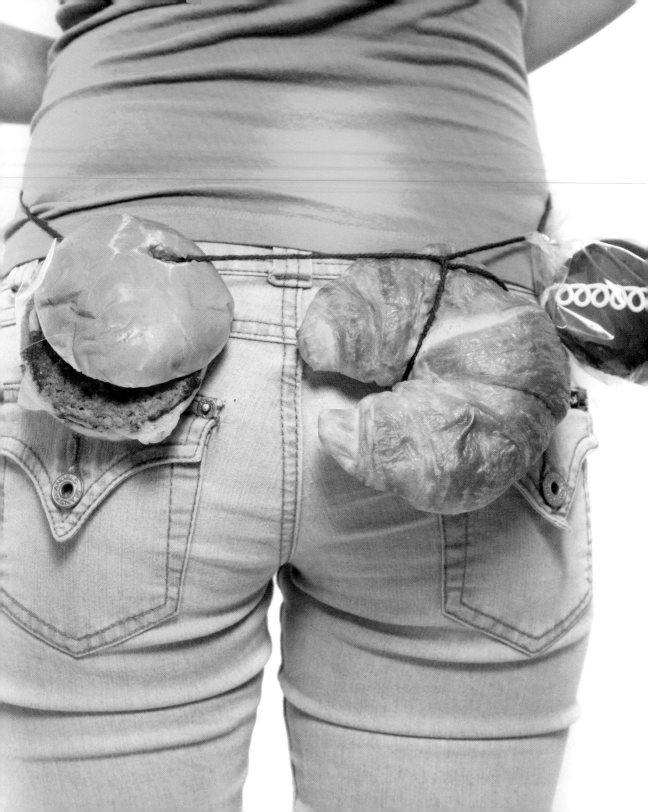

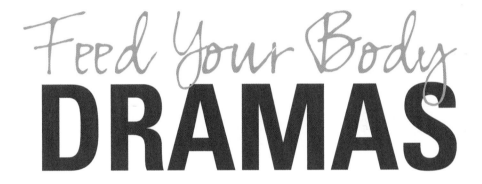

Feed Your Body
DRAMAS

I HATE the taste of healthy food!

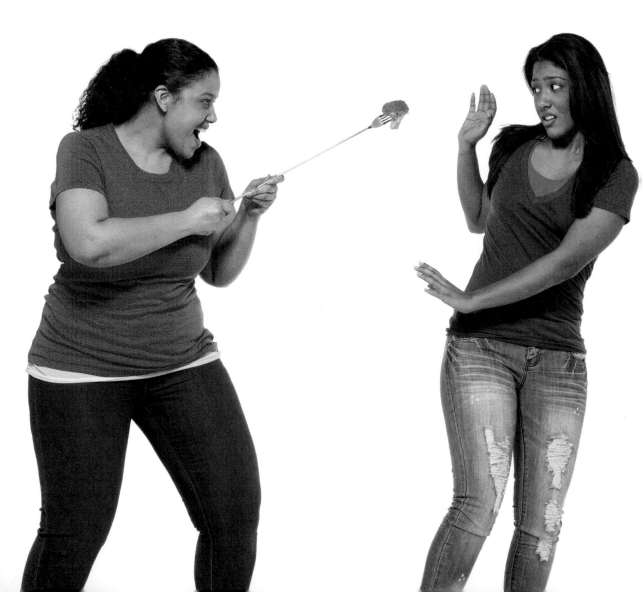

WHAT'S GOING ON?

Admittedly, there *are* only thirty-nine members of the Kale Fan Club (amazingly, the club exists on Facebook), but not all healthy food looks and tastes like rabbit food. What's more, it can be delicious when prepared well. (Kale is good with garlic and onions. Try it sometime!) Still, don't stop reading because you think I'm trying to tell you to throw out everything in your fridge and start growing a garden of green leafies!

Healthy food has gotten a bad rap. Many people don't understand that choosing between "healthy" and "unhealthy" food is relative. Just as having a healthy body is relative to your size, shape, and genetic makeup (a six-foot-two-inch woman can't expect to weigh one hundred twenty pounds and still be healthy), eating healthily starts with looking at what you currently eat and improving upon that first.

HOW DO I DEAL?

First, open your mind to the idea that not all healthy food is disgusting. There are many more tasty, healthy foods out there than you might think, and the common ones you know about are only the tip of the iceberg—and I'm not talking about lettuce. Seriously, how could you not think that pineapple is delicious? (Unless you're allergic, in which case you can substitute cherries, grapes, watermelon . . . the list goes on and on.)

Next, there are no unhealthy foods, only unhealthy portion sizes. Sure, store-bought birthday cake probably contains some trans fats, but if you have one piece at a birthday party, you have little to worry about. If, however, you're eating store-bought baked goods two or three times a week, you may need to reconsider your choices. If you stay within your daily calorie limit and get the proper number of servings from the food groups each day, you can eat just about anything in a reasonable amount!

Here are some ways to improve the health levels of the foods you choose to eat:

☆ Cut the condiments. Sometimes most of the calories in a favorite food come from the stuff we don't care about. Is all that mayo adding anything? Can you taste the added cheese or do you merely like the texture? Does that ice cream sundae taste that much better with loads of whipped cream? Do you need butter on your pancakes or will syrup alone do? Go easy on the condiments and see how many calories you save. If you must drown your food in condiments, hold that mayo, bacon, butter, and cheese, and stick to small portions of ketchup, mustard without the honey, vinegar, hot sauce, and unsweetened relish. Also, ask for them on the side so you can control how much you add.

☆ Make some sneaky substitutions. In a spicy chili, you can hardly tell the difference between ground turkey and ground beef, except for the lack of oil swimming around in it. The same goes for using low-fat yogurt instead of sour cream, trading low-fat milk for full fat, and swapping shredded carrots for shredded cheese on a salad. See what savvy substitutions you can invent!

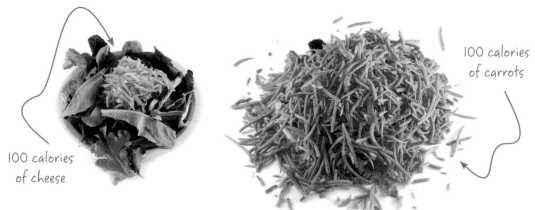

100 calories of carrots

100 calories of cheese

☆ Instead of frying, bake it, roast it, broil it, grill it, or steam it! The oil used to fry a piece of chicken or a slice of potato doubles or triples its calorie count compared to other cooking methods. Add breading and the count goes even higher. The same idea applies to green veggies; steaming preserves nutrients and taste so there's no need to add a lot of butter and salt!

☆ Try new foods twice. Don't knock a healthy food that you think you hate until you try it—twice! Your taste buds may be so out of whack from being coated with preservatives, chemicals, fats, salt, and extra sugars that you need a little time to learn to appreciate a healthy food. Maybe that new food lacks visual appeal because it doesn't resemble a burger and fries, but close your eyes and taste it fairly, and you'll see that it can be yummy. Seriously, once you've made and tasted microwave sweet potato chips (page 200), you may never go back to the potato chip bag again!

Tell If Food Is Healthy

Here's how to tell right away if a food is good for you:

☆ **Did it grow in the ground?** If it's a food that came from the earth and it's for sale in a store, it's probably healthy. Of course you know about berries, fruits, and veggies, but don't forget whole-wheat breads, olive oil, brown rice, oatmeal, and popcorn (without the sugar and butter).

☆ **Does it fly on wings or swim in the ocean?** The right kind of meat is marvelously healthy, too. If it's seafood or poultry, a palm-sized portion is the right amount, as long as it's not fried.

☆ **Is it clear or creamy?** Liquids like soups and sauces that are see-through are often healthier and lower in calories than creamy liquids, except in the case of a sugary soda, which is all empty calories, anyway.

☆ **Does it have a zillion ingredients?** The fewer ingredients, the better, and the fewer ingredients from the fats and empty calories groups, the healthier the food.

☆ **Does it have ingredients that you can't pronounce?** This is a big warning sign. Your best choices are foods containing ingredients that you recognize as real food. Turn to page 216 to learn more about food lingo.

belly laughs

BFF #1: OMG, I love this meal! Can I have the recipe?

BFF #2: Would you believe I got it out of a diet cookbook?

BFF #1: (looking at recipe) Wow, I can't believe it's so good. On paper it looks like it would be gross!

BFF #2: I know. That's why I added butter and cheese and bacon!

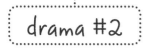
Eating is my hobby. I can't give it up!

WHAT'S GOING ON?

Imagining life without our favorite foods can certainly put the *die* in die-t! Comfort foods earned their name for a reason, and *desserts* can seem to reverse the feelings when we're *stressed*—it's the same word spelled backward! True, you shouldn't bite into a burger just because you're bored but you can still enjoy your favorite foods. In fact, you're more likely

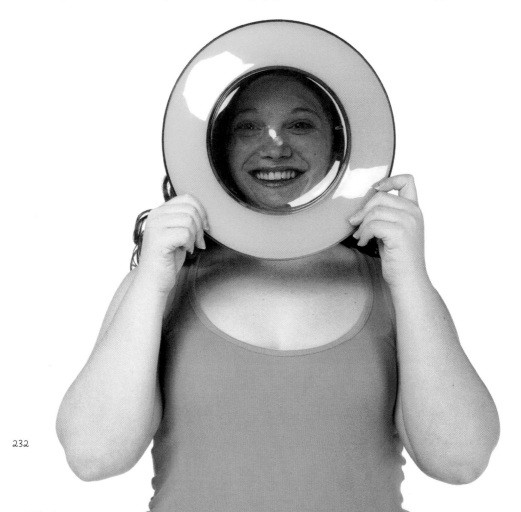

to succeed in healthy eating if you allow yourself some treats. Giving up our favorite foods brings on that feeling of deprivation that can trigger a binge. So relax and enjoy sugary, salty, or creamy treats occasionally. Just try not to go back for seconds . . . or sevenths!

At the same time, try to change how you talk and think about foods. A hobby is an activity you do in your spare time *mostly for pleasure*. While cooking food might fall under this description, *eating food* shouldn't. Noshing on food can be one of the greater joys in life, but food is first and foremost *sustenance*, which is a fancy way of saying that it supports and strengthens the body. Hobbies can be stopped and started at anytime, but food is a requirement for survival. Think about it: Can you swap eating for tennis or knitting? Or could you call breathing a hobby? Or showering? (Don't answer that last one. I don't want to know!)

HOW DO I DEAL?

First things first: Is eating *really* your hobby or is it a way that you deal with stress? Do you eat when you're nervous, bored, or stressed in the same way that some people surf the 'Net or play with their cat when they can't deal with life? If so, find another activity that keeps you sane without snacking. If you find yourself reaching for more ravioli right after dinner, ask yourself if you're hungry or just having a hard time with homework and needing a distraction. If you can't quit hobby eating "cold turkey," try to limit your recreational repasts to a healthy food such as celery or . . . cold turkey!

Second, if you're on a health kick and are trying newer, healthier foods, get used to fueling your body with foods that have not been your favorites in the past. Learn to savor smaller portions and begin to see your favorites as occasional treats, not everyday expectations!

Finally, although eating isn't a hobby, you certainly can enjoy it. Healthy foods might not taste as good to you yet, but give your brain and tongue a chance to adjust! Your emotions have a lot to do with what you enjoy eating, and the happier and healthier you get, the more positive your response to healthy foods will be, so keep an open mind (and mouth)!

fast fact

If you're trying to cover a salad with a teaspoon of dressing, consider mixing the dressing with a little water. It will go farther without adding extra calories!

I can eat healthy for a few days but then I cheat.

WHAT'S GOING ON?

Whether it's a couple of bites of a candy bar or the whole enchilada, "cheating" while on a healthy-eating mission is not like spilling ink on a dress. The stain may ruin your clothes, but nothing can completely ruin your efforts to eat better! Stop thinking of an occasional treat as "cheating." You'll only make yourself feel guilty, which can sabotage your plan for eating well!

HOW DO I DEAL?

Remember, it's all about calories in and calories out. Getting in shape is not a daily tally with a bell ringing and the scale adjusting immediately; the calories consumed and burned over weeks and months are the ones that count. So eating an extra breadstick (even six extra breadsticks) isn't going to ruin your efforts forever. Those extra calories may just slow your progress a little if you're trying to slim down. And as long as you're eating at least 1600 calories a day, you can reduce the impact of the extra calories with extra exercising or by cutting back a little more in the days that follow!

234

Here are some other ways to manage your "cheats":

☆ Cheat once, not always. Splurging once and eating a couple of hundred (or even a couple of thousand) more calories than you should in a day isn't going to keep you from achieving your long-term goals; but doing the same thing three out of seven days in a week will. Calm yourself and get back on track. Overdoing things once or twice doesn't mean you have to make a habit of it.

☆ Don't lie to yourself. If you eat a food, count the calories in it, no matter how bloated the truth makes your daily total look! When you see the caloric consequences of eating an entire pizza written down on paper, you'll know that you want to do better next time—and you won't kid yourself into thinking, "I can't slim down no matter how hard I try."

☆ Plan your "cheats." Look at your schedule and activities. Is your favorite occasion a monthly movie night where you can't say no to melted butter on your popcorn? If a food or event means a lot to you, make room for the extra calories in your schedule and scale back a little on other days to make up the difference!

Dump the Dressing!

f.y.i.

Why cover a 100-calorie salad in 600 calories of dressing, buttered croutons, fried onions, cheese, and bacon? Try these totally delicious salad toppers instead:

☆ **Protein** – mix tuna, chicken, beans, or tofu with your salad veggies for a warm or cold protein punch! This works especially well when the protein source is juicy or marinated!

☆ **Fresh Fruit** – juicy fruits like strawberries, grapes, oranges, are so yummy on salads! When cut up and slightly squeezed, the juice acts as a natural dressing!

☆ **Salsa** – it's the number one condiment in America for a reason. Salsa is delicious with lettuce, tomatoes, cucumbers, and peppers – just hold the cheese (or make it low-fat) and nachos (or make them baked not fried)!

I used to be able to eat anything
and not gain an ounce,
but not anymore!

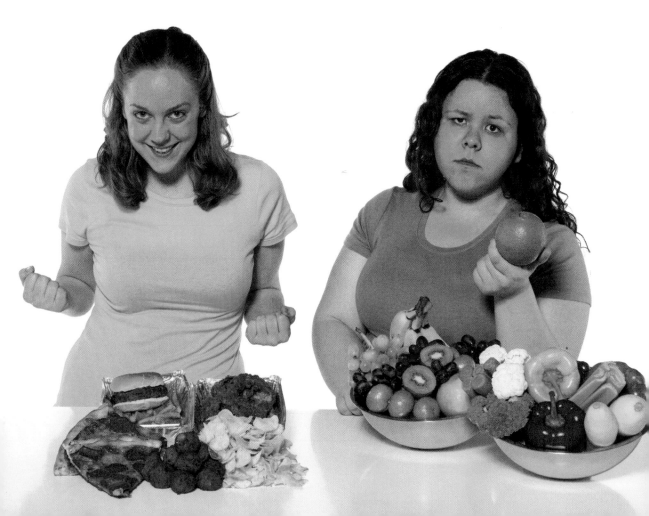

WHAT'S GOING ON?

In your early teens, you probably saw your height change rapidly, or you sprouted an entire size in a month, turning your jeans into capris seemingly overnight. During your growth spurt, which usually happens between the ages of ten and fourteen for girls, your body needs—and burns—a lot of food to keep you growing. But what happens when your hormones pull the plug on puberty and your development starts to slow down? Your body doesn't need as many calories as before, so the food that was being turned into bone and muscle when you were younger now gets stored as fat.

HOW DO I DEAL?

When you're used to eating whatever you want, scaling back can be tough. But before you begin to buckle down to lose weight, make sure that what you're thinking of as extra weight isn't simply normal development. What you might be freaking out about as extra fat may very well be your natural womanly shape. Breasts, hips, thighs, and stomach padding can feel freaky when they first develop—as if they don't belong to you. You may also question how "normal" you are if your body doesn't look "perky" and "perfect" like the models you see in the magazines. Remember: Those pictures are altered by computer programs that erase everything that makes us human! Rounded breasts and dimpled thighs don't mean you are fat or out of shape. These are natural, normal characteristics of a healthy female body.

Having said all that, if you still think you need to slim down, try increasing your exercise level before you cut calories too much. Your body is still growing, and you need good food to build strong tissues and organs. Finally, if you are exercising and eating well, see your doctor if your weight gain continues. You might have a physical reason for weight gain that needs medical attention (see page 57 for more).

BTW:

NO FOOD GROUP IS BAD

Some people who are trying to slim down cut out grains or fats, thinking that those foods are the culprits in their weight gain. That approach is not wise. While some grains and fats are better than others, eliminating the good kinds with the bad hurts you and your health. So instead of giving up certain kinds of foods altogether, choose foods from all the groups and avoid those with minimal nutritional value, such as added sugars and the "bad" fats: cholesterol, saturated fat, and trans fat.

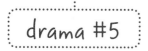

It's HARD to eat healthy around others!

WHAT'S GOING ON?
ZOMIGAWD, it's pizza day and you got a salad?
What are you, on a DIET or something?

> I made your favorite brownies and you're only
> taking a single bite? What an unappreciative
> daughter I have. You usually eat three!

Don't sit next to me with THAT on your tray! Only babies
drink milk. Why didn't you get a soda like always?

> Stop taking yourself so seriously.
> Do you REALLY think that
> one bag of chips is going
> to make a difference?
> Come on, have some!

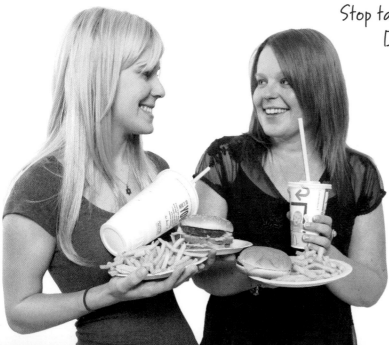

It's difficult enough to try to eat healthily, even when you have lots support from other people. But friends and family frowning on your careful food choices can really put a damper on good decision making! However, before you binge on brownies instead of bananas because you're tired of being bullied, remember what I told you on page 65: when someone teases you, regardless of whether it's about your body type or the food you eat, it is actually a reflection on their issues and insecurities, not yours!

Fortunately, once you tell them about your health goals, most people will start being supportive and will stop belittling your choices (or baking for you). However, it's extremely common for a few friends, and even family, to balk at your new, healthy habits. After all, you're making different choices and altering an eating routine that may have been in place for years! When these people see you taking control of your health and happiness and turning down unhealthy foods that you once enjoyed together, they might react in ways that aren't in your best interest. For example, people who take pride in cooking delicious meals for you often feel unwanted or unloved when you start turning down their food in favor of more nutritious and healthy options. Sometimes they try to make you feel guilty and try to persuade you to eat their food so that they can feel needed and loved. Other people may complain about your choices because your efforts make them painfully aware of how terrible their own habits are. Also, the happier, more confident you that starts to emerge may inspire feelings of confusion, stress, and even jealousy!

fast fact

A recent magazine survey found that 44 percent of young women would order dessert if a friend did, even if they're no longer hungry! The same survey also found that over half of teen girls change their eating habits based on what their friends are chowing down on. This change can be for the better or for the worse, so stay strong and be a positive influence on your friends and help them to change their eating habits for the better, too!

You may be thinking, "Why would anyone be insecure around or jealous of *me*?" Sure, you might be at the very beginning of your journey to health, but every time you make a deliberate choice to get healthy, people notice. That's because, as the rest of this book discusses, when you take care of yourself, the changes affect more than what's on your plate. Your improved eating and exercise habits offer a near-instant boost to your self-esteem, looks, and attitude, too!

HOW DO I DEAL?

People may give you a hard time about your healthy habits, but there will never be a reason good enough to give in and let them interfere with your improvement. If you frequently share

It's one thing to stop sharing meals with unsupportive people, but if you generally feel uncomfortable eating in public and find yourself constantly coming up with excuses to avoid eating where people can see you, tell your doctor or a counselor as soon as possible. One symptom of an eating disorder is frequent reluctance to eat around others. See page 184 for more on eating disorders.

meals with people who constantly comment on your food choices, no matter what is said about your selections or who claims to be hurt by your declining to dine on their delicacies, always remember to:

☆ NEVER give in to the pressure! While you might initially hurt someone's feelings when you turn them down, do you know who gets hurt when you cave and consume the cookies and cakes? YOU! If you have already gently explained to that cook that you're trying to get healthy and are watching what you eat but he or she continues to try to stuff you full, there is absolutely nothing wrong with a firm, polite "NO, THANK YOU!" If the feeder is someone you see often, try to get others to speak up on your behalf also. But always stay strong and steer clear!

☆ NEVER get angry! You are improving yourself inside and out, and getting angry will only set you back. Yelling, returning the teasing, or accusing those who are unsupportive of sabotage will not help the situation or stop the comments. Honest discussions with people about how their comments make you feel can be useful if offered calmly. For example, instead of screaming, "LEAVE ME ALONE!" try sharing, "I know that you love me and are probably just joking, but when you make fun of me for choosing the salad, I feel hurt. Getting healthy is hard for me and I really could use your support." That approach confronts the issue without blaming the teaser.

☆ NEVER lose perspective! While avoiding some negative people may be difficult, especially if they're in your household, keep reminding yourself that for every one person giving you a hard time about getting healthy, there are hundreds, if not thousands, of other people who are cheering you on as you go after and achieve your goals. And that number includes me! Stay focused, and eventually you'll find that many of those who made healthy eating hard for you at first will have become your biggest fans!

I CONFESS:
I GAINED WEIGHT WHILE WRITING THIS BOOK!

That isn't exactly what you expect the author of a book titled **Diet Drama** to confess, right? Let me explain. First, this isn't a diet book. I wrote it not only to give you some facts on food and fitness, but also to start an honest discussion about our health habits, including how hard it is to stay on the good-health bandwagon! For the past eight months, instead of my usual busy schedule spent jetting around the world to speak at colleges and events, I've put in eighteen-hour days at the computer, researching and writing and rewriting (and procrastinating, hee hee). I often felt so glued to my laptop that I wondered if it would take a spatula to unstick me from my sofa!

Needless to say, for a few weeks (OK, for a few months), even my adorable trike collected dust and rust while I put exercise on the back burner to meet my book deadline. After I quickly tired of my slow-cooker concoctions, I admit I turned to frozen dinners for a while and NOT just the healthy ones! I'm not proud of the pounds and pounds that I put on (around twenty!), but I'm not ashamed, either. Weight fluctuations are a part of life, and when they happen, instead of beating yourself up about them, it's best to skip the pity party and get back to being healthy again as soon as you can.

At times in your life, you will gain and lose weight for various reasons: stress, a new relationship (or an end to an old one), a change in your workload, an illness, writing your own book . . . the list could go on and on. A weight change doesn't mean that there's anything wrong with you or that you've "failed." It simply means you are human and your priorities have shifted for a while. As I write this section, my book is nearly complete, but I've decided that I can't wait any longer to start getting rid of this book-induced spare tire. Instead I am literally going out to put air into my tires and take my trike for a spin! Richard Simmons still teaches aerobics class in Los Angeles, and in the morning, I'm going with my girlfriends. His class is a fun and motivational welcome back into the world of working out and watching what I eat! You know what the best thing is about taking a break? When you get back on track, you realize how much better you feel, how well you sleep, and how much more clearly you think. I can't wait to get back into shape and feel great!

HELPFUL WEB SITES *and phone numbers*

EATING AND EXERCISE DISORDERS

National Eating Disorders Association
1-800-931-2237
www.nationaleatingdisorders.org

National Association of Anorexia Nervosa and Associated Disorders
1-630-577-1330
www.anad.org

Overeaters Anonymous
www.oa.org

Binge Eating Disorder Association
www.bedaonline.com

DRUGS AND ALCOHOL

Above the Influence
www.abovetheinfluence.com

Students Against Destructive Decisions
www.sadd.org

National Institute on Drug Abuse
www.nida.nih.gov

Alcoholics Anonymous
www.aa.org

Cocaine Anonymous
www.ca.org

Marijuana Anonymous
www.marijuana-anonymous.org

Narcotics Anonymous
www.na.org

The Cool Spot
www.thecoolspot.gov

National Drug Abuse Hotline
1-800-662-4357

Alcohol Abuse Hotline
1-800-ALCOHOL

MENTAL HEALTH

Mental Health America
www.mentalhealthamerica.net

SUICIDE

American Foundation for Suicide Prevention
www.afsp.org

National Suicide Hopeline
1-800-SUICIDE
www.hopeline.com

BODY IMAGE

Body Positive
www.bodypositive.com

National Association to Advance Fat Acceptance
www.naafaonline.com

NUTRITION

Nutrition.gov
www.nutrition.gov

FOOD ALLERGIES

Food Allergy and Anaphylaxis Network
www.foodallergy.org

Food Allergy News for Kids
www.fankids.org

VEGETARIANS

Vegetarian Resource Group
www.vrg.org

DIABETES

American Diabetes Association
www.diabetes.org
1-800-342-2382

dLife
www.dlife.com

VIOLENCE, SEXUAL HARASSMENT, OR ABUSE

Community United Against Violence
1-415-333-HELP
www.cuav.org

Rape, Abuse and Incest National Network
1-800-656-HOPE
www.rainn.org

National Center for Victims of Crime
1-800-FYI-CALL
www.ncvc.org/

National Domestic Violence Hotline
1-800-799-SAFE
www.ndvh.org

National Teen Dating Abuse Helpline
1-866-331-9474
www.loveisrespect.org

National Child Abuse Hotline
1-800-4-A-CHILD
www.childhelp.org

SMOKING
American Cancer Society
1-877-YES-QUIT or
1-800-QUIT-NOW
www.cancer.org

Nicotine Anonymous
www.nicotine-anonymous.org

SELF-HARM
S.A.F.E. Alternatives
1-800-DONT CUT
www.selfinjury.com

BULLYING
Stop Bullying Now!
stopbullyingnow.hrsa.gov

GASTROINTESTINAL DISORDERS
About Kids GI
www.aboutkidsgi.org

Intestinal Disease Education and Awareness Society
www.ideaskids.com

Celiac Disease Awareness Campaign
www.celiac.nih.gov

GENERAL HEALTH
Center for Young Women's Health
www.youngwomenshealth.org

GirlsHealth.gov
www.girlshealth.gov

PLUS SIZE—FRIENDLY CLOTHING COMPANIES
JCPenney
1-800-322-1189
www.jcp.com

Old Navy
1-800-OLD-NAVY
www.OldNavy.com

Delia's
1-888-533-5427
www.delias.com

Torrid
1-866-867-7431
www.torrid.com

Alight
1-516-367-1095
www.alight.com

b&lu
1-888-992-9899
www.bandlu.com

Fashion Bug
1-866-886-4725
www.fashionbug.com

Lane Bryant
1-866-886-4731
www.lanebryant.com

Sonsi.com
1-866-259-1363
www.sonsi.com

Really Unhelpful Web Sites

The Internet can be a great place to find information on how to improve yourself, but there are also many sites that are full of misleading and dangerous ideas and beliefs, often presented as fact. Steer clear of any site that suggests positivity around behaviors that you know are bad for you, like self-harm, eating disorders, and drugs and alcohol.

f.y.i.

ADDITIONAL RESOURCES

VISIT **WWW.NANCYREDD.COM** TO CONTACT NANCY
AND FOR EVEN MORE INFORMATION, INCLUDING:

- ✰ success stories from more girls in the book
- ✰ delicious, healthy, and cheap recipes
- ✰ calorie counts of common foods
- ✰ online nutrition label resources
- ✰ a comprehensive chart of vitamins and minerals
- ✰ additional exercise resources
- ✰ and much, much more!

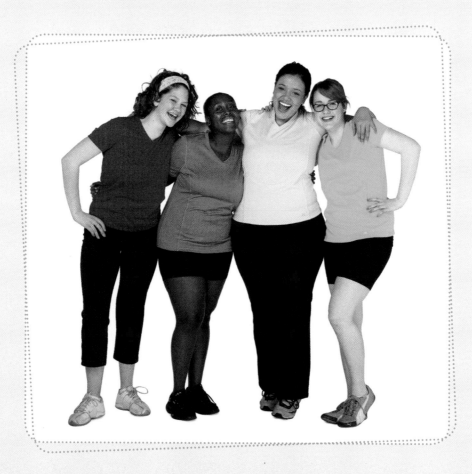

INDEX

Note: Page numbers in *italics* refer to photographs. Page numbers followed by a *tt, fyi* or *btw* refer to text boxes.

ACKNOWLEDGMENTS

Hooray for my hubby, Rupak Ginn, for being the best partner in the world! Also tons of thanks to my mommy, Amanda, my brother, Sammy, my wonderful in-laws, Sunita and Jahar, and Devi, Mallar, and Ishaan and Rishab. I am very lucky to have a fantastic and supportive family!

Casey Hooper, book designer extraordinaire, I could not have done this without you and I'm so grateful for your brilliance and creativity! Also special thanks goes to Jessica Sindler, my talented editor and fabulous friend, you are the best! And to Bill Shinker, Lisa Johnson, and Lindsay Gordon, you and everyone else at Gotham are amazing! Kelly Kline and Katy Bea Martinez-Arizala Keller, you two are phenomenal photographers! And Faith Brynie, how could I ever publish a book without you and your eagle eye? Thanks also to Traci Maynigo for cleaning everything up! Dr. Rome, you have been wonderful to work with—your patients are very lucky! Thanks also to my fantastic literary agents, Todd Shuster and Jennifer Gates of ZSH Literary, as well as Caleb Franklin, Stephanie Paciullo, and everyone else at CAA; you are wonderful! Also thanks to Amy Richards and Jennifer Baumgardner for inspiring me oh so many years ago with your awesomeness!

Further thanks to all my super role models who are featured in this book; Natalie Hodge Cook for everything; Maureen Harrington for her friendship and support; Majora Carter and James Chase; Katy's man Stephen Clifford, Jr., for being fab, and Kelly's assistant Emilee Ramsier, for your talent; Julian Breece and Arianne Cohen for growing up with me and being the best friends a girl could have; the Wine Club Ladies (Gaylyn, Reena, Kim, Missy, Dorothy, Jen, Cecily, Christie, and Marisa) for your support and friendship; style guru Beryl Pleasants for identifying the body types featured in this book; fitness fanatic Michelle Berryhill; Brooklyn Photo for the nightcap and nice studio; Indexing Pros for your talent; Jennifer Monti for introducing me to Dr. Rome; Dr. Hatim Omar for all you do for young people; and early readers Nancy Brown, Ph.D. (special shout out to you from Nancy2!), Leigha Winters, Donna Hunt, and Casey Boykins.

Finally, to my beloved readers and fans, whom I love with all my heart. Always know that you are not alone, and that we are in this together!